DO YOU KNOW . . .

- You can lower your blood pressure with cayenne pepper
- A traditional Chinese physician takes your pulse in twenty-eight places
- Folic acid significantly reduces homocysteine, a toxic amino acid that creates arterial lesions
- Tai chi, the Chinese form of moving meditation, may be the most effective therapy to remove the emotional triggers in a highly stressed person
- Safe plant enzymes found in soy products are more effective than heparin, an anti-coagulant, for improving blood flow through stiff arterial segments
- The homeopathic remedy, natrum muriaticum, can help eliminate edema

PLUS NATURAL ALTERNATIVES FOR CORONARY ARTERY DISEASE, RECOVERY FROM HEART ATTACK, STROKE, HYPERTENSION, CARDIAC ARRHYTHMIA, MITRAL VALVE PROLAPSE, CONGESTIVE HEART FAILURE, AND CONGENITAL DEFECTS

THE DELL NATURAL MEDICINE LIBRARY

PREVENTION, HEALING, SYMPTOM RELIEF . . .
FROM NATURE TO YOU

Also Available from The Dell Natural Medicine Library:

NATURAL MEDICINE FOR BREAST CANCER

NATURAL MEDICINE FOR BACK PAIN

NATURAL MEDICINE FOR ARTHRITIS

NATURAL MEDICINE FOR DIABETES

THE DELL
NATURAL MEDICINE LIBRARY

NATURAL MEDICINE FOR HEART DISEASE

Judith Sachs

Foreword by Martin Milner, N.D.

A Lynn Sonberg Book

A Dell Book

Published by
Dell Publishing
a division of
Bantam Doubleday Dell Publishing Group, Inc.
1540 Broadway
New York, New York 10036

IMPORTANT NOTE: This book was written to provide selected information to the public concerning conventional and alternative medical treatments for heart disease. Research in this field is ongoing and subject to interpretation. Although we have tried to include the most up-to-date and accurate information in this book, there is no guarantee that what we know about this complex subject won't change with time. The reader should bear in mind that this book is not intended to take the place of medical advice from a trained medical professional. Readers are advised to consult a physician or other qualified health professional regarding treatment of all of their health problems. Neither the publisher, the producer, nor the authors take any responsibility for any possible consequences from any treatment, action, or application of medicine or preparation by any person reading or following the information in this book.

ISBN: 0-440-22170-6

Published by arrangement with:
Lynn Sonberg Book Associates
10 West 86 Street
New York, NY 10024

Printed in the United States of America

Published simultaneously in Canada

May 1997

10 9 8 7 6 5 4 3 2 1

OPM

*To a new generation of healthy
hearts, minds, and spirits*

ACKNOWLEDGMENTS

The author wishes to thank Dr. Phillip Bonnet, homeopathic practitioner; Judith Berger, Reiki channel and reflexologist; Pat Chichon, RNC, MSN, PNP, herbalist and alternative health care consultant; and Master FaXiang Hou, Chinese medical practitioner, for their time and guidance.

CONTENTS

FOREWORD

In spite of the amazing strides in drug and surgical intervention in cardiac care, the rate of heart disease in the United States continues to rise. It is the number-one killer of both men and women in America today, and over seventy million are afflicted with some form of cardiovascular illness. The "baby boomers," born between 1945 to 1959, will turn sixty right after the turn of the century. This will greatly increase the numbers of individuals succumbing to heart attacks, atherosclerosis, congestive heart failure, and other cardiac conditions.

Yet much of heart disease is preventable, if not reversible, especially if the patient is willing to integrate conventional medicine with changes in lifestyle and the utilization of natural therapeutics.

In my twelve years of private practice and as a professor teaching naturopathic medical students, I have come to appreciate the subtle responses of the heart to a wide range of influences. First we have genetics, which gives us a base and background for our general health; next, the environment, including allergens and chemical-sensitivity reactions; then prescription medications, alcohol, and other recreational drugs; and last but certainly not least, the emotions, diet, exercise, stress, and mental attitudes about oneself and one's life. These influences play a profound role in the development and evolution of heart disease.

The many and varied facets of an individual's life are all contributing factors that grow and double over upon themselves throughout the decades. And very often the ensuing cardiovascular problems that result are beyond the scope of traditionally trained cardiologists. Even though they may realize that drug therapy or invasive procedures are limited in their ability to heal the heart on their own, they can recommend nothing else. Conventional medical training (and fear of the unknown) leaves out the vast array of lifestyle and natural therapeutic adjunctive care. The patient, too, is often unable to go farther. He or she might say, "I've got a serious condition, and I'd better do just what the doctor ordered." Which in most cases is to keep taking his or her pills and to consider a bypass if the pills don't work.

Certain advanced types of heart disease do require aggressive medical interventions. Yet every type of heart disease can and will benefit from an adjustment of lifestyle and the natural therapies that are outlined in this book. These are well proven in their safety and effectiveness as both an adjunct to conventional treatment and in many cases as an acceptable alternative to a drug regimen that may have many side effects.

In *Natural Medicine for Heart Disease,* Judith Sachs has done a wonderful job of communicating the problems and pathways to success for those who have already been diagnosed with heart disease and those who are perfectly healthy but wish to establish and maintain a preventive lifestyle. She explains the various cardiac conditions as well as practical and beneficial treatments for them. This book educates the reader directly as to how he or she can embrace the best of conventional medicine and integrate it with natural medicine. Both modalities of care, used wisely together, can aid in the management of heart disease and in the development of a true self-care process. The proactive stance of this book shows the reader how best to help heal himself or herself.

Teaching cardiovascular medicine has given me the opportunity to study well the available literature on treating heart disease with natural therapeutics. *Natural Medicine for Heart Disease* is by far the most comprehensive, practical, and easy-to-access book in its class. It is must reading for those who are healthy and want to stay that way, and for anyone with heart disease who is seriously ready to pursue other alternatives to care.

Hold on to your seats and prepare yourself for a new way of health, one that uses all the valuable means at our disposal—allopathic and naturopathic care—to combat heart disease. I wish you the best in your journey in the healing of your heart.

MARTIN MILNER, N.D.
President and Medical Director,
Center for Natural Medicine, Inc., Portland, Oregon
Professor, Cardiovascular and Pulmonary Medicine,
National College of Naturopathic Medicine

CHAPTER ONE

Heart Disease—
An Illness of Body and Mind

Heart disease, the number-one killer of Americans, is eminently *treatable*, and can actually be reversible. If you have no diagnosed disease, you are in an even better position than those who have a cardiac condition, because you can prevent heart disease before it ever develops, even if you have a strong family history of it.

It's pretty common knowledge that we can protect ourselves from cardiovascular illness with nutrition, exercise, and stress reduction techniques. But it's not so commonly known that there is a vast array of other natural remedies—vitamin and mineral supplementation, herbs, homeopathy, yoga, breathing, meditation, biofeedback, and more, that can help you in your quest either to stay free of heart disease or to help treat the cardiac problems with which you've been diagnosed.

We have become so accustomed to the idea of repairing the heart with medicine and surgery that we automatically think of drugs, such as beta-blockers, calcium channel blockers, and clot busters, and high-tech surgical procedures, such as angioplasty and heart bypass, whenever cardiovascular problems are mentioned.

Of course we need conventional medical care to treat heart disease. We are truly fortunate to have a huge arsenal of medical and surgical therapy at our disposal, since so many of us are afflicted. Over seventy million Americans have some form of cardiovascular disease, be it hypertension, coronary artery disease, stroke, arrhythmias, rheumatic heart disease, or congestive heart failure. Although we used to think of heart disease as a man's problem, this is by no means the case—both men and women suffer from cardiovascular illness. Typically men start experiencing symptoms in their early to late forties, and women join them in their late fifties and sixties. Of all those afflicted, nearly one million die each year.

Evidently we need every means at our disposal to combat this killer—so we must have more ways to deal with heart disease than are offered by Western medical science alone. Fortunately we can combine our reliance on medication and surgery with a wide range of complementary therapies that are less expensive, noninvasive, and, when used appropriately, have no side effects. These holistic medical treatments include nutrition, vitamin and mineral supplementation, stress management, herbs, homeopathy, mind-body therapies, Chinese and Ayurvedic medicine, and other treatments such as biofeedback, chelation therapy, Reiki, and reflexology.

These treatments for heart disease do not replace but rather *complement* the conventional medical care you will be receiving from your general practitioner or cardiologist. The therapeutic techniques allow your system to reach its optimum level, where it can make the best use of the medicines, diagnostic procedures, and surgeries you might have. Complementary care is both preventive and restorative—it heals not just the body but the mind and spirit as well, so that it can actually make you want to live longer and in better health.

How to Use This Book

Always consult your primary health care professional before beginning any complementary therapy. It's a good idea to bring this book with you to your doctor's office so that the two of you can go over the possibilities for adjunct care and decide which holistic treatments would benefit you the most.

In order to receive excellent health care, you must know how to ask informed questions. So before you make any choices about which therapies to use, you'll need to read chapter 2 in order to understand the nature of heart disease and also to grasp the basics of the various complementary treatments. You will also learn the conventional medical approaches for each cardiac condition.

Next, because you need a thorough grounding in good preventive health care, we'll plot out an easy-to-manage program of diet, exercise, lifestyle changes, and stress reduction that will make it more feasible for you to start taking charge of your heart health. Whether you have already been diagnosed with heart disease or are simply concerned about keeping your healthy heart in the best shape possible, you need to use the information contained in these chapters and make them a continuing part of your general health plan.

Next, we outline the various complementary therapies. These include separate chapters on the basics and use of mind-body practices such as meditation, yoga, and tai chi chuan; supplementation; herbalism; homeopathy; Chinese and Ayurvedic (Indian) medicine; and finally, biofeedback, chelation therapy, Reiki, and reflexology.

You will not necessarily wish to use every modality of treatment described in this book—nor do you need to. But it will be important to learn which therapies might be right for you and to use them, with your doctor's knowledge and approval, in conjunction with your conventional medical care.

How do you make such a decision? Begin with a therapy that interests you enough so that you will stick with it for a period of months. Complementary therapies do not work overnight, and require persistence for maximum benefit. If your doctor has said that your main problem is the need to lower stress, for example, you'll have to make time each day for your new yoga and meditation practice. If you are at a stage in your medical therapy where you must stay on a strict drug regimen but wish to help your body and mind to enhance what medication can do, you might try Reiki or reflexology. And if you are a basically healthy individual with a strong family history of heart disease, then a combination of herbal medicine, homeopathy, tai chi, and biofeedback might work in tandem to reduce your risk factors.

This book will act as a guide to a new appreciation of health options. The ultimate decision as to what choices to make should be based on your awareness of how you react to new ideas and new situations.

The Difference Between Curing and Healing

When we think about using natural therapies to improve the condition of someone with heart disease or to prevent heart disease from developing in the first place, we're not looking for a "cure." Nutrition, herbs, homeopathy, Chinese and Ayurvedic medicine, and mind-body techniques will make a positive difference in the general good health of the individual rather than targeting the heart and "fixing" the problem. These therapies may also improve certain symptoms, such as an irregular heartbeat or high blood pressure or high cholesterol. But more importantly, they will make a substantial change in the way we care for ourselves and in the way our body and mind respond to that care.

Medical and surgical specialists practice the art and science of dealing with *dis-ease,* something that literally makes the body uncomfortable or dysfunctional. In the medical view an organ or tissue must be targeted for surgical "renovation" so that the body can be "cured," or restored to normalcy.

But as we know from the hundreds of thousands of heart disease sufferers who undergo surgical procedures and are continually medicated, a cure is very rare. Many individuals survive for years after a heart attack or bypass as mere shadows of their former selves, too weak and debilitated to live full, vital lives.

In the holistic view, on the other hand, the sick organ or tissue is simply a sign that the whole person is out of harmony or balance. It is therefore useless to treat just the heart, since every system contributes to this imbalance. We must identify the underlying causes of disease in the mind, the spirit, and the emotions as well as the body before real change can be expected.

How Western Medicine and Holistic Therapy View Heart Disease

Let us examine the case of Matthew, a forty-five-year-old vice president in a Chicago advertising firm. He is slightly overweight; eats a diet heavy in red meat and dairy products and light in vegetables, fruit, and fiber; spends an occasional Sunday morning on his rider mower; and rarely has the time to exercise. He is a classic "type A" personality—quick to anger, impatient with subordinates, a half-a-pack-a-day smoker who pops a beer or two when he gets home from work each night. He is divorced, with two children in college. Every time Matthew gets angry, a vein pulses in his forehead. He is winded when he climbs stairs or sprints to catch a bus, and sometimes he has a feeling like a knife stabbing his chest that truly alarms him. Because these pains always stopped as soon as he sat down and rested, he neglected to make regular medical appointments over the years. It's only recently, due to his girlfriend's insistence, that he decided to seek some professional advice about his heart.

Treatment by Traditional Western Medicine

Matthew's doctor ordered an electrocardiogram to check his heart's pace and rhythm, did a battery of blood tests, and did several blood pressure checks, some at rest and some during an exercise stress test. He diagnosed Matthew as having angina, a symptom of his coronary artery disease, hypertension (high blood pressure), hypercholesterolemia (high cholesterol levels), and a slightly enlarged heart.

He put Matthew on a diuretic (Hydrodiuril) to reduce blood and fluid volume and thereby lower blood pressure, as well as a beta-blocker (Tenormin) to slow his heart rate and reduce pressure in blood vessel walls. Even though the drugs gave him a dry mouth, made him feel dizzy, and took away his sex drive, Matthew understood that these were necessary to his treatment. His doctor also suggested that he take off some weight, cut down on the smoking and drinking, and try to control his anger better.

In order to find new ways to manage Matthew's stress that would work in conjunction with the medication he was taking, Matthew's physician approved his patient's decision to consult with several different holistic practitioners. Matthew would not necessarily follow each course of therapy recommended (herbs and conventional medication might counteract each other, for example), but he made appointments with quite a few practitioners to see what they would each recommend. Matthew wanted options that he'd never tried before in order to break some of his long-standing habits and felt that the focus of trying one or two of these new therapies would keep him on track. After he had visited all the practitioners, he and his physician would decide which would work best for his condition.

Treatment by Holistic Practitioners

Matthew saw a homeopathic doctor, who, in addition to a physical exam and blood tests, did a lengthy interview to gain information about Matthew's past, his preferences, his behaviors, and his current lifestyle. He felt that Matthew's personality was one that lent itself to patterns of overeating, constipation, and shortness of breath. These attributes are typical of a person with an imbalanced calcium metabolism. The remedy *Calcarea* would be prescribed in a high dosage, *Natrum mur*, to control his blood pressure, and *Aconite* at the beginning of the treatment to reduce panic and calm Matthew down. He also gave Matthew specifics about a low-fat, high-fiber diet, swimming as well as daily stretching exercises, a smoking-cessation program, and an ongoing stress reduction regimen that included meditation and yoga.

The herbalist Matthew saw asked him to change his diet considerably, reducing his salt intake and eliminating all meats and rich sauces. She also counseled him to cut out smoking and alcohol and start a regular program of swimming and gardening. Her herbal prescription included hawthorn to improve blood supply to the heart; dandelion root as a diuretic that would help reduce his blood pressure and also act as a tonic to the whole body; dandelion leaf as a diuretic; with plenty of additional potassium and lime blossom to dilate the peripheral blood vessels and relax the whole body.

The Chinese medical doctor saw Matthew's problem as an imbalance between his liver and his kidney, where the *yang* (or forceful nature) of the liver is excessive and *yin* (or receptive nature) of the kidney is deficient. In addition to recommending several Chinese herbs, the doctor performed acupuncture on various points on the Liver and Kidney meridians (see chapter 8 for an explanation) as well as points on the Gallbladder and Bladder meridians. He counseled Matthew to lose weight and avoid alcohol and tobacco, and eliminate sweet and fatty foods from his diet. He also counseled him to do only gentle tai chi exercises so as not to overexert himself.

The difference between the various therapies as opposed to Western medicine should be clear: The allopathic physician is using drugs to affect the heart and the various tissues that affect heart function; the holistic therapists are examining the total person and finding areas that need strengthening so that the heart *and every other organ and tissue* can flourish. And both means of care can work together to create a generally healthier individual.

Men and Women and Heart Disease: Understanding Your Risks

There are a variety of risk factors for heart disease—some which can't be changed and some which can. The more categories that pertain to you, the greater your risk of contracting heart disease. And this means that the more risks you can avoid or reduce, the healthier you'll be in the long run. Because holistic treatment concentrates on the entire person rather than just the heart, you will be working to eliminate many of these risks simultaneously.

Risk Factors You Cannot Control
Gender: Men have a greater risk of suffering a heart attack than women below the age of fifty-five. Being a woman and producing the hormone estrogen (which keeps your good cholesterol high and your bad cholesterol low) reduces your risk of heart disease in your reproductive years. However, after menopause, when you lose the protective buffer of es-

trogen, your risk rises to equal that of men. Rising levels of stored iron after menopause (not lost as it used to be during menses) may further increase a woman's risk.

Age: Four out of five heart attack victims are above the age of sixty-five. As they age, women are twice as likely as men to die within a few weeks of a heart attack.

Family history: If you have one or more immediate family members who had heart disease or a heart attack below the age of forty (for men) or fifty-five (for women), you are at higher risk yourself.

Race: African-Americans, Hispanics, and some Native Americans tend to have more risk factors than Caucasians. In particular African-Americans tend to have high blood pressure twice as often as Caucasians and severe hypertension three times as often.

Risk Factors You Can Control or Manage

Smoking: If you smoke, your risk of a heart attack is more than twice that of a nonsmoker. In addition, smokers who have a heart attack are more likely to die within an hour of the attack. Nicotine raises blood pressure; toxins damage artery walls. Smoking can also lead to blood clots and constricted blood vessels in legs, kidney, heart, and brain. Secondhand smoke is also a danger—the risk of death is increased by 30 percent if you're exposed to someone else's smoking habit. But if you quit, your risk rapidly recedes until, fifteen years after you stopped smoking, your risk just about equals that of a person who's never smoked.

Cholesterol levels: Cholesterol, a type of fat the body produces and that we also ingest when we eat foods that have fat in them, comes in two varieties. HDLs (high-density lipoproteins) are the "good" cholesterol that keep plaque deposits off our arteries. Our HDL level should be higher than 45. LDLs (low-density lipoproteins) are the bad cholesterol that help to create deposits of plaque, which can block arteries.

Our LDL level should be lower than 130. The surgeon general's recommendation is that total cholesterol level should be less than 200; however, statistics show that lowering the level to 150 is a surer guarantee of never having a heart attack.

If your total is above 240, your risk of heart disease doubles. In order to lower your levels, you *must* maintain a diet low in fat—especially saturated fat—and a program of daily exercise. There are, however, people who produce higher amounts of cholesterol in their liver, and it's very difficult for them to achieve the recommended levels by dietary means alone. Natural therapies often offer a variety of ways to lower cholesterol without medication.

Triglycerides: Triglycerides, another form of fat produced by the body, are not in themselves independent risk factors for heart disease, but they are particularly significant in women. Your triglyceride level should be below 130, something that can be achieved by diet, exercise, and natural therapies.

Weight: You should not be more than 20 percent over desired weight as determined by life insurance tables (see pages 71 and 72 for an appropriate weight table). Even if you have no other risk factors for heart disease, obesity makes you more likely to develop heart disease and stroke. Too much weight taxes the heart and makes it work harder than it should. It also influences blood pressure and cholesterol and can lead to diabetes.

Hypertension: When the pressure under which the blood is pumped through your circulatory system is too high, it increases the heart's workload, eventually enlarging and weakening the heart muscle. Blood pressure tends to increase with age but can be managed with diet, exercise, restricted sodium, and the natural therapies outlined in this book. Your systolic pressure (the top number) should be under 140; diastolic pressure (the bottom number) should be under 90.

Diabetes: The disease known as diabetes mellitus interferes with the body's ability to balance blood sugar levels and can also lower HDL cholesterol. Obesity makes you more likely to develop diabetes, and having diabetes in turn increases your risk of higher blood pressure, kidney disease, blindness, and nerve and blood vessel damage. (Since you may have a genetic predisposition to this disease, it is not always a controllable factor, but it can be managed.)

Stress: Feeling pressured and overwhelmed produces adrenal hormones (adrenaline, noradrenaline, and cortisol) that may trigger arrhythmias (irregular heartbeats) and raise blood pressure. Many researchers think that the increase in pressure may also break down the lining of the blood vessels, allowing plaque to be deposited there.

Alcohol: A little bit of alcohol (between 4 and 6 ounces of wine a day) is beneficial to the heart, because it has been shown to raise HDL levels. However, as soon as you go slightly above this amount, the tide turns the other way. Alcohol abuse can lead to liver damage, mental disorders, accidents, and injury and may fill the body with toxins that damage the heart and blood vessels. Many natural and Eastern therapies prohibit the use of alcohol completely.

Social isolation: Individuals who are isolated have more difficulty taking care of themselves physically and finding the emotional impetus to get well and stay well. It's been found that cardiovascular health (and health in general) is improved when a person has a support system in place.

Social status: Poor, uneducated individuals tend to know less about health care and may not be able to afford the services of medical professionals. If they have heart disease, it may go undiagnosed and over the years may worsen from neglect.

When you look at heart disease from a holistic perspective, you will understand that many factors—some physical, some psychological, some social—make you more or less susceptible to getting ill. Although you are handed certain factors you cannot change, you can make enough of a difference in the factors that are under your control to alter radically your chances of staying well. The more risk factors you moderate or eliminate, the better your chances of good health.

It's been clearly shown that preventive care makes a difference—if you change certain elements in your life, you can avoid heart attacks or chronic heart disease.

Finding the Right Doctor or Health Care Practitioner

If you have already been diagnosed with heart disease or have suffered a heart attack, you are undoubtedly under the care of a cardiologist or family practitioner. *Be sure to continue to see your physician regularly and follow all of his or her recommendations.*

At the same time, however, you can benefit your own treatment by expanding your horizons and consulting practitioners of natural medicine. This is equally true if you don't currently have heart disease but know that you have a family history of it, or fall into one or several of the risk categories mentioned above.

Being Truthful with Your Physician

It is not always easy to approach a medical professional with a concept of multidisciplinary holistic care. And many individuals have found that they are ridiculed by their primary-care physician when they say they want to visit an herbalist, a homeopath, a nutritionist, or a naturopathic physician.

However, if you have decided that natural healing is what you want, you should not lie to your physician about it. If you are on high blood pressure medication, for example, you should be forthcoming with information about any supplemental, herbal, or homeopathic preparations you are taking or about exercise programs you wish to start. You should list everything you are taking and doing—be accurate about the brands and dosages of vitamin and mineral supplements, herbs, and homeopathic remedies—to make sure that you can combine them with the drugs you are taking, that there are no contraindications, and that your dosages are within a safe range. Remember that not all complementary treatments are completely benign, and some may need careful monitoring when taken in addition to medication.

Make your doctor a partner in your overall care. You may find that he or she is more than a little interested in the fact that your blood pressure and cholesterol levels have dropped dramatically since you started eating differently, meditating, and practicing tai chi. If you don't regard the person in the white coat as some supreme authority, but rather as a guide to better health care, your chances for a good outcome will improve immediately.

If your physician is totally opposed to your wish to expand your health care horizons, it's possible you need to consult a naturopathic or holistic physician who specializes in cardiac care.

Where to Find Complementary Therapists

How do you find experienced, competent practitioners in the various natural therapies? Use the Resource Guide in chapter 11 to direct you to organizations that can refer you to a holistic practitioner. A holistic medical center is your best bet for "one-stop shopping" when it comes to complementary therapies. You may find holistic centers listed in your Yellow Pages under "Health Care" or "Health Services." These centers usually combine the best diagnostic services with an array of different specialists in complementary treatments. You can also ask any therapist you're interviewing for names and numbers of other clients or patients.

How to Determine If This Is the Right Therapist for You

Pay attention to the way the therapist responds to you. Remember, you are a paying customer and you deserve good service. Is he or she a good listener? Does he answer the questions you've asked or admit he doesn't know but will try to find an answer? Do you feel comfortable about the way he or she examines you? Think about the ways in which he asks you to do certain things—to move, to cough, to undress for further examination. He should still be attentive to your needs even while he assesses your condition.

Be as specific as you can when talking about your pain (where it is, what it feels like, how often you experience it, what makes it better or worse, how long you've been having this type of pain), shortness of breath, nausea, palpitations, or any other symptoms you've noticed. You should tell your holistic practitioner which medications you take, what your diet and exercise program are like (honestly!), and how you currently handle the stress in your life. Go over all your concerns in detail—you may want to write them down before you see the therapist so that you'll remember everything.

Be sure that you understand the diagnosis and recommendations for treatment. If you don't know why you should be having a certain test or taking a certain remedy or herb, ask. If this practitioner feels there is something you've been doing that could be harmful, make sure you understand why. If you wish to stop taking a medication that a medical doctor has prescribed for you, you may need to wean yourself off it slowly and only under your doctor's and holistic practitioner's supervision.

Be wary of therapists who insist that they can "cure" you, or that you will need years of treatment before you see a change in your heart condition. It is true that most natural or complementary therapies work in a cumulative fashion—the more you stick to the healthy programs you've instituted, the better you'll feel. But there is no guarantee that you will undergo a miraculous recovery with complementary care or that you won't have a heart attack or need surgery somewhere down the line.

If you have decided to consult more than one therapist as well as your primary-care physician, make sure you know how your doctor will communicate with the other individuals you're seeing. Encourage practitioners to report to each other about your health status.

Be sure you understand the way your therapist handles payment. Most insurance companies do not reimburse you for alternative or complementary care; however, there are some new insurance programs (see Resource Guide, chapter 11) that offer coverage if you qualify for their plans. Since you will have to pay most of your own bills up front, you should arrange a payment schedule with the therapist, and be certain to discuss a time in the future when you will begin to reduce the frequency of your visits.

The heart has enormous potential. If we care for it well, we can keep it beating soundly throughout our long lives.

CHAPTER TWO

Treating the Heart's Problems

Before there was a pill to lower cholesterol or a tiny balloon to insert inside an artery, there were herbs and nutritive foods that could change the chemistry of the blood. There were meditative and energetic techniques to quiet the mind and the sympathetic nervous system, curtailing the destructive stress response that might lead to a heart attack.

Always consult your primary-care physician before embarking on any new therapies. Never alter your dosages or medications without the express agreement of your doctor.

In order to use natural methods to help heal the heart in an appropriate and safe manner, we must first know some facts about the heart and the cardiovascular system. This chapter will reveal the workings of the heart and arteries and will detail the medical and surgical therapies that are currently being used in allopathic care. Finally, it will describe how the different types of natural medicine can complement conventional medical and surgical care. And armed with this information, whether you are interested in prevention or you've been diagnosed with heart disease and are already undergoing conventional medical treatments, you will be able to make sound judgments about ways in which you can use natural medicine to improve your heart health.

How Does the Heart Work?

The human heart is a hollow, muscular pump that moves blood throughout your body from birth to death. It starts beating about twenty days after conception and keeps going for seventy or eighty years or more. It is the core of the circulation system, moving blood around your body and back again, mixing it with oxygen and supplying the various organs and tissues with the nourishment they need to survive and function.

The body contains sixteen pints of blood, and each day the pump recycles them a thousand times. During an average lifetime the heart pumps 1.8 million barrels of blood through the body.

The heart is apportioned into four chambers and is divided down the center by a partition called the *septum*. The right *atrium* (top right side) receives the unoxygenated blood returning from the veins in the rest of the body and delivers it to the *right ventricle* (bottom right side), which pumps the blood into the lungs, where it is mixed with oxygen. The *left atrium* (top left side) then receives the oxygenated blood and delivers it to the *left ventricle* (bottom left side), where it is then pumped out to the rest of the body through the arteries.

The opening from atrium to ventricle is known as a *valve,* which is a one-way mechanism for blood to flow through the heart.

The heart receives its own blood supply from the three coronary arteries: right main, left main (with its branch known as the left circumflex), and the anterior descending.

The various problems that affect the heart may have to do with lessened capacity, malfunctions, or overcompensation, when the heart is forced to work too hard and becomes

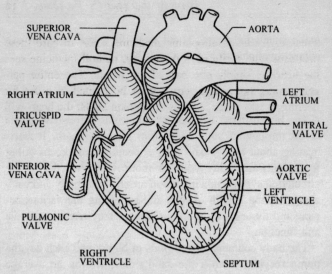

THE HEART AND ITS VALVES

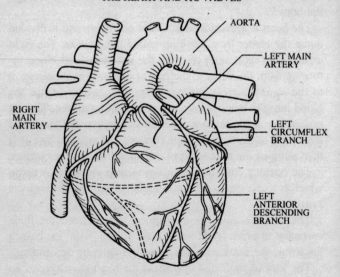

THE CORONARY ARTERIES

stressed. Although allopathic medicine seeks to cure these problems with medication or surgery, natural medicine sees the heart as simply one part of the whole. The entire person—mind, body, and spirit—must be treated in order for healing to take place. And as the person heals, the heart will too.

How Do You Know If Your Heart Is in Good Shape?

Every American is at risk for heart disease. Unlike conditions such as malaria or tuberculosis, you don't have to be exposed to a parasite or a bacterium to come down with a "disease of affluence." Although there are of course genetic factors and family predispositions to cardiac problems, the majority of illnesses having to do with the heart are caused by lifestyle—too much rich, fatty food; too little exercise; too much stress; not enough attention paid to preventive health care, good diagnosis, and time for healing pursuits such as meditation and breathing.

What brings on heart disease? Surely the slow buildup of cholesterol that causes plaque to block coronary arteries is a major factor. But there are other problems that reduce the flow of blood to the heart: Blood platelet aggregation causing a clot that can block an artery is extremely dangerous, as is arterial spasm, where a sudden "cramp" torques a coronary artery, shutting down the oxygen and blood supply. Major stresses in our lives cause the release of the "fight or flight" hormones, which also affect the proper functioning of the heart and cardiovascular system.

And the problems begin at a very young age. Autopsies done on children as young as three years old showed that plaque had already started to damage their tiny arteries—so you can imagine what your arteries might look like at thirty, forty, or fifty.

This doesn't mean that you can't change your heart health! With the proper attention to good preventive care and use of the healing arts described in this book, you can make a huge difference in the future of your heart—even if you have already suffered a heart attack or undergone angioplasty or bypass surgery. But you have to work at it.

First you must have a checkup by an experienced professional. If you are already under medical care for a heart condition, you are undoubtedly being monitored and should continue to see your physician on a regular basis. But if you are currently healthy and are interested in preserving your heart, here's what to do:

- Get a thorough wellness exam so that you can find out what your risk for heart disease is. (See chapter 1 on "Finding the Right Doctor or Health Care Practitioner.") You will need a family history, if possible, and a written list of what you typically eat over the course of one week, your exercise program, and those elements in your life that cause you stress and how you deal with them.
- Your health care practitioner will give you a complete examination, including a medical history, a profile of your heart risk, a good diet and exercise plan, and suggestions for treatments—allopathic and complementary—that are right for you.
- You will need blood work—a cholesterol profile including your LDLs, HDLs, and total cholesterol level; triglycerides; and blood glucose levels.
- You should have several blood pressure readings taken. A newer method to ascertain your risk of heart disease and stroke involves first a measurement of the difference of pressure in your arms and ankles, then a noninvasive acoustic test (Doppler) that measures narrowing of the carotid arteries that carry blood to the brain. In a study

of 5,200 older adults at four sites across the country, the duplex scanner was able to show blockages in the arteries that feed the brain before any real damage had occurred. The arm-to-ankle blood pressure measurement is a very telling figure—in perfectly healthy individuals the measurement is the same or similar; in those with extensive atherosclerosis the ankle reading is low (indicating that the heart is having a problem moving blood against the force of gravity to and from distant sites in the body).

- An EKG (electrocardiogram) should be performed to get a baseline picture of your heart patterns. The lines or waves that appear on the readout show the electrical activity of your atria and ventricles. From this test a physician can see the heart rhythm, any enlargement of one or more chambers of the heart, and any injury to the heart muscle or old scarring from a previous heart attack.

  If you have already been diagnosed with heart disease or have had a heart attack or undergone surgical treatment for a cardiac condition, you should also have the following tests:

- An exercise stress test, or a treadmill test with thallium (a radioactive dye injected into your arteries). During this test, as you walk on a treadmill and are hooked up to an EKG, your physician can see how your heart rate and blood pressure function when your body is working hard. The thallium test shows whether all areas of the heart are getting enough blood.

- An echocardiogram, so that your physician can see a picture of the structure of the heart created by the sound waves reflected from the heart. In this test you lie on a table and a transducer wand is passed over your body. A three-dimensional image of your heart then shows up on a screen.

What Can Go Wrong with the Heart?

The major problems of heart disease are the following:

Coronary Artery Disease (CAD, or atherosclerosis)

Symptoms: Angina (pain), shortness of breath, blackouts or fainting, palpitations, great fatigue.

Possible traumatic events: Heart attack, stroke.

CAD is caused by a loss of oxygen and nutrients to the heart muscle because of diminished blood flow. Atherosclerosis, the development of plaques that narrow and eventually block the arteries and reduce the volume of blood flowing through them, is the most common form of coronary artery disease.

As there is increasingly less elasticity in the arteries, it becomes harder for oxygenated blood to flow through them, and slowly the supply may be cut off to the heart and other organs. If a piece of plaque ruptures, a blood clot *(occlusion),* can form and completely block the artery. If the vessel narrows completely and closes up, or a blood clot breaks loose elsewhere in the body and travels to the heart, where it creates a blockage, you may suffer a *myocardial infarction,* or a heart attack (see page 26). In rare cases an attack may also be caused by an *arterial spasm,* where a sudden cramp shuts off blood flow. A *stroke* occurs when the arteries to the brain are blocked.

The most classic symptom of CAD is *angina,* a crushing or squeezing pain in the center of the chest, which often radiates out to the jaw, left arm, or shoulder blade. It is sometimes accompanied by nausea, fainting, sweating, and cool, clammy extremities. The episodes of terrible pain generally stop when you sit or lie down. (There are two other forms of angina, *unstable angina,* which increases in frequency and duration and is not alleviated by rest; and

Prinzmetal's angina, which is usually caused by an arterial spasm.)

Conventional treatments: The goal of medical treatment is to increase the supply of oxgyen to the arteries or reduce the heart's demand for oxygen. A physician will diagnose coronary artery disease by listening to your description of symptoms and then performing the tests described on page 21, sometimes repeating them a year or so after you have been on medication.

MEDICATION

Nitrates are the first line of treatment for anginal pain in the form of the medication nitroglycerine, a vasodilator that opens up the blood vessels.

Diuretics remove water and salt from the body so that blood volume goes down and the heart doesn't have to work as hard; that is, blood pressure falls. Unfortunately, diuretics may raise cholesterol (a major cause of CAD) and blood sugar levels. When water is removed from the body, valuable minerals are also washed away, and the loss of potassium may leave you feeling weak and fatigued.

Beta-adrenergic receptor blockers block the stress hormones (adrenaline and noradrenaline) that can make arteries constrict. They slow down the heart and reduce blood pressure. But they can also slow things down too much, causing incredible exhaustion in many patients and an impairment of heart rhythm. These drugs have also been shown to reduce libido and cause major sexual dysfunction, particularly in men. Your physician must wean you off these drugs *very* slowly because a rapid withdrawal can cause a myocardial infarction.

Angiotensin inhibitors (ACE inhibitors) block the reaction of a particular enzyme that causes smooth muscle to constrict or narrow. These drugs, too, have side effects—some patients get severe allergic reactions.

Calcium channel blockers are drugs that treat hypertension and coronary artery disease, which have a direct effect on calcium ions, which constrict cells and narrow arteries. The drugs block calcium ions from entering cells, so that the vessels can dilate and blood pressure can drop. These drugs are also used to treat arrhythmias and hypertension (which may lead to or coexist with coronary artery disease).

Aspirin thins the blood and thus makes it less likely that clots will form. Studies on men have found that an aspirin a day is a good preventive tool against heart attacks. (It is assumed that the same medication in the same dosage will be effective with women; however, there have not as yet been clinical trials to prove this.)

Hormone replacement therapy (HRT) (for women only). A controversy rages as to whether replacing the estrogen and progesterone that women lose at menopause with synthetic hormones will prevent heart attacks and ward off other forms of heart disease. Because estrogen keeps the protective HDLs high and LDLs low, HRT is often prescribed, particularly for women with a strong family history of heart disease, or those who've already had a heart attack. However, in order to maintain the protective benefit of these hormones, only long-term therapy will do—and more than five years on HRT has shown to increase risk factors for breast and endometrial cancers.

If medication has not alleviated the symptoms of coronary artery disease, you may be told that some type of invasive procedure is the next step.

INVASIVE PROCEDURES

Cardiac catheterization or angiogram is the gold standard of cardiac diagnosis. In this test a catheter is inserted in a vein in the arm or groin and snaked into the heart to determine the amount of blockage in the coronary arteries. If it is significant, a balloon angioplasty will be recommended.

Angioplasty (PTCA, or percutaneous transluminal coronary angioplasty) is a procedure in which a small balloon is introduced at the end of the catheter and inflated when it reaches the site of blockage. The pressure of the balloon's opening presses the destructive plaque to either side of the artery wall, thereby opening a passage for blood to course through.

Bypass surgery (CABG, or coronary artery bypass grafting) When the coronary arteries have become so blocked by plaque that they no longer carry the blood efficiently enough around the heart and back out to the rest of the body, and if angioplasty has failed to keep the arteries open, conventional Western medical thought is that bypass surgery is the necessary next step. This operation involves taking a vein from the leg or chest and creating a diversion for the blood supply, similar to a detour on a major highway that bypasses the congested traffic. The extremely expensive bypass operation should be performed only on those with severe angina, left main-vessel disease, and some categories of heart disease that affect all three coronary arteries at once.

After bypass a person must stay on medication and radically reduce dietary, stress, and lifestyle excesses. Even then most patients generally only enjoy five to seven relatively healthy years before new plaques have formed and either another angioplasty or another bypass is needed.

Directional atherectomy is a procedure in which a tool with a rotating cutter with a diamond tip, similar to a tiny drill, is introduced via a catheter into the artery to cut away the plaque. It has been found that this procedure is less effective and often more dangerous than traditional balloon angioplasty.

Laser ablation or laser with balloon angioplasty is an experimental technique being used only in research settings. In this procedure a laser beam is directed at the area of blockage and aimed to remove the plaque. It has also been tested in conjunction with balloon angioplasty. However, neither use of the laser seems very promising in cardiac therapy, and its results indicate that it may not make it into general clinical use.

Myocardial Infarction

Symptoms: searing, crushing, strangling pain mid-chest, often radiating out to the left arm; nausea and vomiting; diaphoresis (cold sweat); shortness of breath; a feeling of foreboding and doom.

If coronary artery disease is so advanced that the heart muscle cannot receive sufficient blood supply, a heart attack (myocardial infarction) can occur. As the insides of the arteries harden with plaque, it becomes increasingly difficult for the heart to get all the blood it needs. This condition is known as *ischemia.* If a plaque has completely blocked an artery leading to the heart (an *occlusion),* this can cause a heart attack. Men and postmenopausal women are the prime candidates for this cardiac event. Although it's quite common for many people to relegate the pain of angina to "indigestion," for most individuals who experience the most exquisite pain of a lifetime, it's hard to deny a heart attack.

But there are also "silent," asymptomatic heart attacks. The condition known as *silent ischemia* can be more dangerous than the type that announces its presence with angina. In this case, the heart isn't getting enough oxygen, but the only way it can be spotted is on an electrocardiogram. This type of heart disease will show the same abnormalities on this diagnostic test as it would if the patient had angina. The need for early detection is vital.

Conventional treatments:

MEDICATION

Nitrates are the first line of treatment for anginal pain in the form of the medication nitroglycerine, a vasodilator that opens up the vessels.

Clot busters such as tPA (transplasminogen activator) can be used with certain patients to thin the blood dramatically within a couple of hours after an attack. Heparin (another blood thinner) may also be given the following day.

Antiarrhythmic medication, such as Lidocaine, is used to keep the heart rhythm normal.

Cardiotonic drugs, such as digitalis, are used to slow the contraction of the heart muscle, increasing cardiac output and helping to get fluid out of body tissues.

ACE inhibitors get the heart pumping more efficiently.

Beta-blockers control the sympathetic nervous system response.

Calcium channel blockers control arterial spasm and lower blood pressure.

Morphine is used for pain and sedation.

INVASIVE PROCEDURES

PCTA (see page 25), and if necessary, CABG (see page 25.)

Stroke

Symptoms: Weakness and numbness in the limbs, face, or down one side of the body; inability to speak or understand others; one-sided blindness (sudden onset); dizziness or falling; loss of consciousness.

When blood flow cannot reach the brain, a stroke will occur. Very often a plaque breaks off and travels through the body until it arrives at the brain (a *cerebral embolism),* or possibly a blood vessel in the brain ruptures (a *cerebral hemorrhage).* This causes the death or damage of thousands of brain cells, many of which affect motor abilities.

Conventional treatment: Physical and speech rehabilitation, at least three times a week soon after the event, for up to a year. A true desire to be functional again is practically a necessity to recovery.

Hypertension

Symptoms: Sometimes none; sometimes headache or shortness of breath.

A normal blood pressure, as set by the National Institutes of Health, should be no more than 140/90. The top figure (systolic) is measured when the heart contracts and pushes blood into the artery; the bottom figure (diastolic) is the pressure in the arteries when the heart muscle relaxes in between beats.

When blood pressure is elevated, the heart is forced to work harder in each contraction and relaxes under higher pressure in between beats. By working harder, it increases the force of the blood pushed against the arterial walls, which can damage them. Someone with hypertension may have thickened and enlarged heart walls. Heart failure can result. The kidneys and the eyes can also be damaged by hypertension.

In a hypertensive individual, blood has to travel through the arteries at high pressure, something like a high pressure hose with a powerful spray as opposed to a garden hose where the water simply flows through. High pressure can damage arterial walls. The heart has to work harder and use more oxygen to get the blood to circulate. As the insides of the arteries become coated with plaque, atherosclerosis may develop.

If the arteries are rigid and narrowed by plaque, they will put up resistance to this high pressure blood flow. In doing so, the heart walls will thicken and dilate. Eventually heart failure may result.

Conventional treatments:

MEDICATION

ACE inhibitors, calcium channel blockers, alpha- or **beta-blockers,** and **diuretics.**

LIFESTYLE
Low-sodium diet.

Cardiac Arrhythmias

Symptoms: Palpitations, tachycardia, brachycardia, irregular heartbeats.

Although there are designated areas in the heart that are responsible for establishing and maintaining the beat, other areas in the atria and ventricles also have the capacity to generate an electrical impulse. If one of these impulses interrupts the ordinary rhythm of the heartbeat, this can set off an irregular heartbeat—an *arrhythmia.* If the normal rhythm is disrupted for a prolonged time, *fibrillation* can result.

Atrial fibrillation occurs when the walls of the upper chambers of the heart contract in a rapid, nonrhythmic beat, as many as 300 beats a minute. This may occur after a heart attack, during an anginal attack, or to people who have congestive heart failure, or atherosclerosis.

Ventricular fibrillation occurs in the lower chambers of the heart and prevents blood from flowing out to the rest of the body. The patient may have no pulse and may stop breathing, requiring emergency CPR and defibrillation. This is a very dangerous situation, which can result in death.

PAT, or *paroxysmal atrial tachycardia,* happens when the atria contract at a very fast rate and the ventricles respond as well, creating an overall fast heartbeat.

Brachycardia, or *brachyarrhythmias,* occur when the atria contract too slowly and the ventricles respond. If the heartbeat can't rise above the 40s and the least exertion causes shortness of breath, the condition is known as *heartblock.*

Conventional treatments:
MEDICATION

Antiarrhythmia medications come in four classes. One makes the heart less excitable, the next (beta-blockers) blocks production of stress hormones by the sympathetic nervous system, the third slows the heart's cells as they return to their resting state after a beat, and the fourth causes the heart to beat less forcefully. All of these drugs are powerful and can cause serious side effects if not dosed precisely for the patient's needs. You must be monitored by your physician when you first take these drugs. These medications are used for patients with *tachycardia,* or an excessively fast heart rhythm only.

INVASIVE TECHNIQUES

Artificial pacemakers take over the job of producing electrical impulses for the heart. These are implanted in a pocket created under the skin on the chest. They are *essential* for patients with brachycardia who have uncontrolled second- and third-degree heartblocks.

AICD (automatic implantable cardioverter defibrillator) shocks the heart back into a normal pattern whenever an arrhythmia occurs. It is implanted in the abdominal cavity.

Mitral Valve Prolapse

Symptoms: There are often no symptoms, but a physician may be able to hear a murmur or "click" on examination with a stethoscope. Many cases go undiagnosed until midlife, when shortness of breath and arrhythmias may develop. Some people develop a brief stabbing chest pain (different from anginal pain) to the left of the breastbone that occurs at intervals, as well as palpitations, dizziness, numbness, arrhythmias, and fatigue.

This disorder seems to run in families and is much more common in women. When the mitral valve is prolapsed, it becomes enlarged and floppy. It doesn't snap closed when blood leaves the left atrium—instead the leaflets billow out and blood can leak backward into the atrium, causing the classic "click" followed by a murmur.

This condition is not life-threatening, although the onset of symptoms sometimes makes patients anxious or panicky. The only real danger is that it predisposes many to bacterial endocarditis, an inflammation of the lining of the heart's membranes.

Conventional treatments:
DIAGNOSTIC PROCEDURES
  Echocardiogram.

MEDICATION
For those with chest pain, **beta-blockers** or **calcium channel blockers.** **Antibiotics** should be given before dental work and surgeries or certain procedures as a prophylactic against endocarditis.

Congestive Heart Failure

Symptoms: Shortness of breath (often waking a person from sleep with a feeling that he or she is suffocating), coughing or wheezing, rapid heartbeat, great fatigue, swelling—especially in the legs and/or abdomen and chest.

This condition results when the left ventricle cannot pump the amount of blood the body needs. Pressure then mounts in the pulmonary veins, and fluid collects in the lungs and legs, bringing on shortness of breath and fluid retention, which causes the body to swell. As the heart tries to accommodate to the increased pressure on the lungs, the left ventricle cavity dilates and the muscle is "stretched," enlarging the heart. This syndrome is serious and may be predictive of a shortened life span. Very often patients with congestive heart failure have other cardiac problems (tachycardia, hypertension, valve disease) that complicate the medical picture.

With congestive heart failure the body retains water from reduced cardiac ouput, resulting in swelling of body tissues. This increases the workload of the heart even as it is losing its ability to pump and contract efficiently. When the heart can't keep up with the body's demands, the individual feels terribly tired and weakened.

Hospitalization is often required to take immediate measures to get water and salt out of the body. In any case a patient with congestive heart failure must be monitored closely by a physician.

Conventional treatments:
MEDICATION

Digoxin (Lanoxin), a derivative of digitalis, to stimulate the contractile ability of the heart.

Diuretics (Lasix) to lower fluid retention and reduce the edema (swelling).

ACE inhibitors (Vasotec) to widen blood vessels so that the heart won't have as much trouble pumping blood through them.

Congenital Defects

Symptoms of pulmonary stenosis: Shortness of breath.

Symptoms of aortic stenosis: Angina, fainting, heart failure.

Symptoms of shunt malformation: Murmur, shortness of breath.

If certain structures don't form correctly in utero, or don't align properly before birth, you may be born with a particular abnormality or malfunction. Most congenital heart defects are not life-threatening and need no treatment. But others, those that cause obstructions or impair the passage of blood flow, may cause symptoms. If symptoms appear, the usual course of action is to repair the defect surgically.

Any one of the four valves can develop problems, either through congenital defects, coronary heart disease, or the aging process in general. A valve may develop *stenosis,* where it becomes narrowed and its leaflets don't open and shut properly. A valve can become *leaky* and permit blood to flow in the wrong direction—this is most typical of the mitral valve, where *mitral regurgitation* is a common problem. Any valvular disorder puts a burden on the heart, which compensates by becoming enlarged and weakened.

Conventional treatments:

Treatment for any malformations due to obstructions (stenosis or a narrowed pulmonary or aortic valve):

INVASIVE PROCEDURES

Balloon valvuloplasty, a technique similar to angioplasty (see page 25) will widen the narrowed valve.

Treatment for **left-to-right shunt malformations** (atrial or ventricular septal defects that leave an opening between the two sides of the heart):

Repair of opening, or **catheter closing** of some atrial defects.

How Natural Medicine Can Assist the Body in Its Healing Process

Heart disease is an extremely serious condition and must be diagnosed by a medical professional. But even if you are currently under a doctor's care and taking medication, this does not mean that you can't help yourself in other ways at the same time. This is equally true if you are not ill but are deeply concerned with maintaining or improving your heart health.

Natural remedies can work directly to reduce coronary artery disease, hypertension, high cholesterol levels, arrhythmias, and congestive heart failure, and can be of great benefit in the prevention of and recovery from stroke. They will not have any direct effect on congenital heart problems or heart valve disease; however, some of these defects are associated with nutritional deficiencies—particularly CoQ10 and magnesium. Natural medicine and good nutrition can help the status of the heart, even if surgery is necessary as well. In addition, an overall holistic care program will support and strengthen all the systems of the body so that it will respond faster and more effectively when treated with allopathic medicine.

The following complementary therapies will be discussed fully in subsequent chapters. But it is important that you familiarize yourself with them first, so that you know which direction to take when you are considering holistic care.

NUTRITION

What you eat may be the prime influence on the condition of your arteries and heart. Therefore you should maintain a low-fat, low-sodium, high-fiber diet to prevent or recover from heart disease. Saturated fat encourages the body to produce cholesterol, which ends up as plaque on the arteries. The American Heart Association recommends that you reduce your intake of fat to between 20 to 30 percent of your total caloric intake. (Most Americans consume about 37 to 40 percent of their calories in fat.) However, in order to reverse heart disease, it's been shown that you must get down to 10 percent.

EXERCISE

In study after study vigorous daily activity has been shown to lower blood pressure, improve cardiac function, lower blood glucose, reduce the blood's tendency to form clots, burn off body fat, eliminate leg cramps, and do wonders to increase HDL cholesterol and decrease LDL cholesterol. Even for those who've already suffered a heart attack, this therapy is beneficial. In an evaluation of more than four thousand heart attack survivors, it was found that exercise rehabilitation programs produced a 25 percent reduction in second attacks and the overall death rate.

Aerobic exercise, anaerobic exercise (that which uses the body's resistance against gravity), and flexibility and endurance training are all essential facets of a well-rounded exercise program.

SUPPLEMENTATION

Although we get vitamins and minerals in our food, in order to improve our heart health, we need higher amounts of certain nutrients than occur in a normal diet. In a ten-year study on the benefits of supplementation of over eleven thousand individuals at UCLA, survival rates from heart disease in those who took five to ten times the RDA for vitamin C were 42 percent better for men and 30 percent better for women. Similar studies exist for vitamin E, which has been shown in tests on laboratory animals to help prevent heart attacks. Studies on individuals who consume supplemental vitamins and "quasi"-vitamins, minerals, fatty acids, amino acids, and trace elements (vitamin A, CoQ10, vitamin B_6; selenium, zinc, manganese, L-carnitine, SOD, lysine, pycnogenol, EFAs, and EPA) are quite compelling. Most of the data indicate that symptoms for coronary artery disease, hypertension, arrhythmias, valve disorders, and congestive heart failure are reduced more effectively with supplementation than without it.

STRESS MANAGEMENT

The more stress we succumb to, the more stress hormones we produce. These in turn elevate LDL cholesterol levels and allow negative changes to take place in the blood vessels, narrowing and hardening the arteries.

One of the goals of stress management is to give individuals the control they need over such emotional reactions as anger, fear, depression, and so on, which trigger sympathetic nervous system responses. Through a wide variety of techniques—from breathing and meditation, to time management, goal setting, and behavior modification—stress can be dealt with and used for positive rather than negative outcomes.

MIND-BODY APPROACHES

In order to manage stress, it is necessary to practice a type of therapy that will help us to relax. The two most widely practiced forms of mind-body therapies are yoga, an ancient Indian series of postures combined with breathing, and tai chi chuan, an ancient Chinese system of moving postures combined with breathing. Meditation is an integral part of both disciplines. Dr. Dean Ornish, of the Preventive Medicine Research Institute in California; Jon Kabat-Zinn, Ph.D., of the Stress Reduction Clinic at the University of Massachusetts Medical Center; and Dr. Martin Milner, of the Center for Natural Medicine in Portland, Oregon, all prescribe mind-body therapies as stress reduction tools and give convincing evidence that these healing arts lower blood pressure and heart rate and supply better blood flow throughout the body.

HERBAL MEDICINE

There are many specific herbs that have been known to have a healing effect on the heart; however, their action may take a long time, especially if used in lower doses, and work best in combination with an excellent diet. Certain herbs (hawthorn, lime blossom, dandelion root and leaf, garlic, valerian, cactus, convallaria, coleus root, and parsley) are effective in treating coronary artery disease, hypertension, arrhythmia, congestive heart failure, and valve disorders. They can be taken in the form of infusions, decoctions, tinctures, extracts, tablets, capsules, and pressed juices.

HOMEOPATHY

Homeopathic remedies are diluted doses of natural elements that cause the same symptoms as a particular illness. (See chapter 7 for a complete explanation of homeopathy.) The theory behind this treatment is that "like cures like," or a little bit of something that might make you sick encourages the body to rally its own energies and fight the disease. Homeopathic remedies may be so diluted as to contain infinitesimal amounts or even none of the original substance; however, the energetic remnant of that substance is what triggers the body's own healing ability. Particular remedies are not just symptom-based but are also personality-based—different types of individuals will take different remedies for hypertension, anginal pain, coronary artery disease, congestive heart failure, and arrhythmias.

CHINESE MEDICINE

(See also chapter 8.) The guiding principles of this ancient healing tradition are *yin* and *yang*. *Yin* represents everything in life that is yielding, soft, dark, receptive, feminine, and water-based. *Yang* includes all elements that are strong, forceful, light, active, and fire-based. The two are not considered opposites, but rather two unified sides of the same coin. If the body is sick, this is because a pattern of disharmony exists that has disturbed the balance of yin and yang.

In order to make a diagnosis and decide on treatment, a practitioner of Chinese medicine also refers to the twelve major meridians, or lines of energy, which connect along a succession of specific points throughout the body. Complete therapy would include acupuncture (treatment with fine needles to access energy along different meridians), herbal therapy (Chinese herbs specific to heart ailments, such as ginseng, Tang-Kuei formula, Bupleurum, Dragon Bone Combination, and coptis), as well as *qi gong,* or directed breathing techniques.

AYURVEDIC MEDICINE

The word means "the science of prolonged life," in Sanskrit, and the principles by which this type of Indian medicine is practiced involve preventive care, healing, and a philosophy of living. Everything that affects your heart will have either a positive or a negative effect on it—the hours you work, the foods you eat, the scents you wear. The three mind-body types are crucial to any diagnosis. *Pitta* tends to correspond to our type-A personality, and is a fiery, strong-willed, impulsive individual who might suffer from coronary artery disease. *Vata* tends to be spiritual and creative but often very anxious and might be prone to mitral valve prolapse or arrhythmias. *Kapha* tends to be physically heavier, rather lethargic, and hard to motivate. This person might be predisposed to diabetes or congestive heart failure. An Ayurvedic doctor would prescribe changes in diet, exercise, warm oil massages for stress, and herbal tinctures for these various cardiac conditions.

BIOFEEDBACK

This technique uses a machine to teach you how to alter your normally involuntary bodily functions, such as blood pressure and pulse. A trained practitioner will show you how to use relaxation techniques in conjunction with information about your body's physical responses. During the sessions, sensors running from a biofeedback machine are attached to your skin, and the readouts appear on the machine's meter. When you are under stress, your readings will be significantly higher than when you are able to control your breathing and use your mind to lower your blood pressure.

CHELATION

This treatment for atherosclerosis involves a washing of the narrow, blocked arteries with certain agents (an amino acid called ethylenediaminetetraacetic acid—EDTA, the anticoagulant heparin, the mineral magnesium, vitamin C, and several other vitamins) in order to remove calcium and other harmful minerals from the blood. Getting rid of abnormal deposits via this intravenous drip allows a restoration of blood and oxygen flow throughout the body. Chelation is reputed to dissolve arterial plaques so that they can be flushed out through the kidneys in the urine. Another mechanism in this process involves the formation of collateral blood vessels, which can actually take over for damaged ones if necessary. The treatment is approved as a standard treatment for lead poisoning, but is not accepted by medical practitioners as a treatment for coronary artery disease. But it is on the FDA's GRAS (Generally Recognized as Safe) list.

ENERGETIC APPROACHES

The following two therapies use the energy of the body to heal itself. Reiki, a Japanese therapeutic touch therapy, channels healing energy to the heart. The practitioner will hold his or her hands over the various parts of the body in order to bring energy to the affected area. This is a good additional complementary therapy that can help to speed healing of all the body systems.

Reflexology is based on the belief that specific areas in the foot correspond to different internal organs and that by pressing on these various areas, you can help to heal the organs. The point coresponding to the heart is thought to be located on the left foot, halfway across the pad under the toes, approximately under the break between the second and third toe. Although a reflexologist would work on areas of the foot that correspond to the entire body, the most direct method of working on someone with CAD, hypertension, or irregular heart rhythms would be to stimulate this heart point. The therapist would also work on the head reflexes (located on the tips of the toes) to be certain that the brain-heart connection was strong in order to prevent a stroke or heal complications arising from a stroke.

Controversial Therapies That May Need More Research

There are many authoritative studies that validate all of the complementary treatments listed above—often the scientific proof of their worth is equal to that of conventional medical treatments. No form of medicine is foolproof. Sometimes, regardless of years of clinical trials, there can be disasters—thalidomide and DES, for example, were drugs that were insufficiently tested and caused serious problems when placed too quickly on the open market. Similarly, natural medicine has many therapies without sufficient research to warrant general use right now.

Most of the therapies discussed in this book have been practiced for centuries, and are often credited even by conservative physicians. For others, with fewer studies to their credit, it may be more difficult to substantiate their beneficial results. Although it is relatively easy to find anecdotal evidence of positive results, you should be wary of therapies that promise too much.

HYPERBARIC OXYGEN THERAPY

This controversial therapy requires the patient to sit for a couple of hours in a sealed chamber at twice the normal atmospheric pressure while breathing pure oxygen through a mask. The goal is to increase oxygen in the bloodstream so that it can act as a natural "free-radical" scavenger and heal the arteries and other heart and brain tissue. Those who feel that more research is necessary dispute the speed with which the body gets more oxygen during this therapy. The procedure delivers and disseminates O_2 quickly. Plaque deposits take a very long time to dissolve, and the oxygen may not have enough time to work before dissipating in the tissues.

Although it is not harmful, it is still unclear as to whether this therapy really works for heart disease.

OZONE (O_3)

In this technique, blood is drawn from the patient, mixed with ozone, and then delivered back to the patient intravenously. It is used widely in Europe, but there are only a few doctors using it in the United States. The procedure is said to increase the oxygen content of the blood similar to hyperbaric oxygen therapy. Unfortunately O_3 supplies the body with O_2 plus an extra oxygen ion, which is spun off as a free radical. There is potential for therapeutic use of oxygen delivered orally and intravenously (after being mixed with the patient's blood); however, as yet we don't have sufficient evidence of its value in cardiac care.

FASTING

This extreme form of dietary therapy, even under supervision, can be very dangerous. The goal of therapy is to remove toxins from the body (most recommended fasts don't last much beyond four days). However, for a person weakened by heart disease, the drop in blood sugar and blood pressure from a total lack of nutrients can be exceedingly harmful.

DIAPULSE

This is a technique in which the patient is hooked up to a machine that delivers electromagnetic waves into the bloodstream. This creates a "cellular massage." It is said to increase blood circulation to the tissues, open the arteries and veins, and remove waste matter that causes inflammation and swelling. This technique is often used to accelerate wound healing; however, it is not approved as a therapy for atherosclerosis. Like oxygen therapies, although it poses no danger, it may not be effective.

The Best Care for Your Heart

When you care about your good health, you want to explore all possible avenues of healing. Some—such as eating right and making sure you get your body moving energetically each day—are very familiar. Others clearly have merit, because of their foundation in reasonable thinking or because they've been around for thousands of years. You may feel that some other treatments are not substantially researched, or you may find that they simply don't work for you.

In a well-rounded holistic healing program, many different techniques and therapies combine to renovate and activate your mind, body, and spirit. Of course your primary-care physician is your first stop on the road to good health. After the two of you have agreed on your basic treatment, you can start to use the chapters that follow as a guide to maintaining, preserving, and improving your heart.

CHAPTER THREE

The Three Golden Rules
of Preventive Heart Care

It's so simple. You have only three golden rules to remember if you want to stop heart disease in its tracks and stay healthy. If you follow these simple guidelines, your risk of heart disease will plummet. And even if you have already had a heart attack or undergone bypass surgery, you can repair a great deal of damage simply by obeying the golden rules.

RULE ONE: Eat in moderation, less than you think you need. Make sure your diet is extremely low in fat, animal protein, sugar, and salt; and high in fiber, carbohydrates, and soy products.

RULE TWO: Make an unbreakable commitment to exercise moderately every day. A brisk two-mile walk will do, but you can add swimming, biking, hiking, and dancing if you like.

RULE THREE: Keep your lifestyle on an even keel. Stop smoking for good, and reduce the amount of caffeine and alcohol you currently consume. Get at least seven hours' sleep.

These three rules are the best insurance you can have against heart disease and may help you in reversing the condition if you've already been diagnosed with it. By changing your habits *just a little,* you can make the biggest difference in your health and avoid the need for medication or surgery. You can also start to feel better than you ever have, which will keep your commitment to these three rules strong. As you work on your holistic program of preventing heart disease, you'll find that it's no longer work, but simply an enjoyable way of life.

Nutrition—Your Best Defense Against Disease

If there is one change you could make today that would improve your cardiovascular profile, it is the food you consume each day. If you have already suffered a heart attack or undergone bypass surgery, you *must* make the commitment to a different type of eating if you are not to re-create the situation that caused your disease in the first place. If you don't go right to the core of the problem and resolve it, your bypass will clog up just as your coronary arteries did initially.

Dr. Dean Ornish, a pioneer in cardiovascular care from the Preventive Medicine Research Institute in San Francisco, California, has shown that a plant-based, low-cholesterol diet combined with daily exercise and stress management can eradicate blockages in blood vessels and keep them clear. His patients, many of whom had arteries that had been blocked for years, are a testimony to the fact that human effort and simple, safe therapies that involve the most basic elements can save lives.

Dr. Ornish looked at the general American diet and the recommendations for altering it and decided that a much more radical change was in order. Most of us consume from 37 to 40 percent of our daily calories in fat, and many people are up at the 50 to 60 percent level. Foods high in saturated fat are often high in cholesterol, which invades the blood vessels and leads to the accumulation of plaque. In a traditional "healthful" eating plan, Dr. Ornish noted, doctors were telling patients to reduce their fat consumption to 20 or 25 percent daily. But he found through his work on thousands of patients that in order to reverse heart disease, nothing less than 10 percent will do. (Dr. Nathan Pritikin, of the Pritikin Center at Duke University School of Medicine, actually advocated this type of diet for the prevention and treatment of heart disease as long as fifteen years ago.)

And the benefits you gain from healthy eating go way beyond preventing a heart attack. A diet that protects your heart will

- fill you with energy and well-being
- improve your body image as you see your shape changing to match your excellent eating habits
- motivate you to stick with an exercise program that will make you hungry for more good food

Controlling Your Weight

Obesity is a significant risk factor for heart disease and stroke, so it's important that you maintain a weight that's within 20 percent of what's recommended by insurance companies. If you're carrying a lot of extra pounds, you're making your heart work harder each time it beats. Obesity influences blood pressure and cholesterol levels and also predisposes you to diabetes.

It's preferable of course to keep setting new weight goals as you lose very slowly—about half a pound a week is the healthiest way to go. After you're at your 20 percent mark, you can aim for a 10 percent mark.

The perennial question, How do you lose weight sensibly and keep it off? is actually not such a difficult one if you're committed to a heart-healthy nutrition program. If you do switch from being a carnivore to a vegetarian who only occasionally dabbles in very small portions of meat, fish, chicken, or turkey, *you will lose weight without drastically restricting calories.*

If you are very dedicated and committed to preventing heart disease or preventing a recurrence, you will live by the one basic maxim:

EAT NOTHING THAT WALKS, SWIMS, FLIES, OR CRAWLS.

If you avoid all food that comes from animals, you cannot go wrong. By drastically reducing your fat intake, you will automatically lower your cholesterol and blood pressure. The elimination of animal foods, including dairy products, will cleanse your whole system, as well as strengthening and supporting your heart. A plant-based diet, filled with luscious vegetables, grains, and fruits, can give you a brand-new life with a brand-new heart.

On the other hand if you are a die-hard carnivore, making dramatic changes may not be a good idea, because you will fall off the wagon, give yourself a lot of guilt and stress, and perhaps end up with more erratic and harmful eating habits than you had before. If you're the type of person who cannot do without hamburgers or chicken wings, ask your doctor whether you might keep animal foods in your diet if you drastically reduce the amount you eat. By limiting yourself to four ounces of animal products daily, you can stay sane and healthy too.

There are many exciting foods on the market that are good for your heart that you may never have tasted. The more experimental you are in your adventures with vegetables, soy products, and some ethnic foods, the more varied your healthful diet will be.

Working Your Way—Slowly—Toward Good Nutrition

Don't attempt to make radical changes in your diet all at once, and be sure to sit down with your health care provider to discuss the changes you'd like to make. I suggest that you start out with a diet of roughly 1,800 to 2,000 calories a day, with a 25 percent fat content (450 to 500 fat calories a day) and work your way down slowly to 12 or 10 percent. Make sure you include foods that you really like in addition to trying new foods. If you're squeamish about vegetables, remember that *everything* tastes good when cooked in a little olive oil and garlic. If you've never tried legumes, *every* bean tastes wonderful when simmered with a bay leaf, thyme, and a pinch of salt and pepper. And grains such as kasha, couscous, amaranth, and brown rice are uniformly excellent when cooked with some onion and low-salt vegetable broth.

Over time, by eliminating foods that are detrimental to your health and substituting foods that care for your heart, you will find that eating is more pleasurable as well as more healthful.

Changing the American Food Pyramid

The U.S. Department of Agriculture food pyramid has been touted as correct eating for most Americans. It does suggest a well-balanced diet that includes all food groups, heavy on the bottom with carbohydrates, vegetables, and fruits, and light on top with animal products, dairy, fats, oils, and sweets. However, the recommendations of this pyramid are for a diet that takes 30 percent of its calories from fat, which is much too high if you want to make a real difference in your cardiovascular health. So we will have to shave off the top where the animal products live, flattening out the pyramid into a trapezoid.

* * *

Here is the adapted version of a good eating plan:

BREAD, CEREAL, RICE, AND PASTA: 6 to 11 servings daily (one serving is 1 slice or ½ cup).

VEGETABLE GROUP: 3 to 5 servings of ½ cup daily.

FRUIT GROUP: 2 to 4 servings of ½ cup daily.

SOY PRODUCTS (see page 50 for a discussion of the new importance of soy to cardiovascular health): 2 to 3 servings daily, equaling from 25 to 50 grams (this includes tofu, tempeh, miso, and commercial products such as "No-Dogs"). Soy products are *not* low in fat; however, they encourage the production of HDL cholesterol in the blood.

LEGUMES: 1 serving daily, ½ to 1 cup.

MILK, YOGURT, CHEESE GROUP: 1 serving daily, 1 cup each, low-fat varieties. Only skim or 1% milk and no-fat yogurt. Soy cheese is an acceptable substitute for animal cheese. The lowest-fat animal cheese is Parmesan (which you'll use less of anyway, since you only sprinkle it on your food).

MEAT, POULTRY, FISH: 2 to 3 times a week only. A meat, poultry, and fish serving is 3 to 4 ounces. It can be used as a "condiment" in vegetable dishes or stir-fries.

EGGS, NUTS: to be consumed very rarely, once every other week or two, or according to your doctor's recommendation. Egg is preferably only egg white or one whole; nuts, approximately ten.

FATS, OILS, SWEETS GROUP: use sparingly. Best to restrict this group to 1 tablespoon of olive or canola oil for cooking. See page 49 for alternative suggestions to fats.

A Healthy Heart Diet Means Low Fat Plus Low Cholesterol

Before you can get your cholesterol levels on an even keel, with your HDLs ideally ranging between 45 and 65 and your LDLs below 130, you must first regulate the amount and type of fat you eat. Fats are carbon and hydrogen atoms joined into structures called *fatty acids*.

Saturated fats, which are solid at room temperature, such as butter, lard, and the fat on meat and poultry, are the culprits that create havoc in our arteries. They raise the levels of bad cholesterol (low-density lipoproteins, or LDLs) and stimulate the liver to produce its own cholesterol and deliver it to the bloodstream.

Unsaturated fats come in two varieties. The good ones (monounsaturated) are olive oil, canola oil, and the omega-3 fatty acids, which you get in cold-water fish. These will bring down your LDL cholesterol while leaving your HDLs intact. But the polyunsaturated vegetable oils, such as margarine, have been partially hydrogenated so that they can stand up on a piece of bread. These fats are just about as bad for your health as butter, because the hydrogenation process creates trans-fatty acids that raise LDL cholesterol levels and also lower HDL cholesterol levels. (Other nonhydrogenated oils like safflower are in a liquid state and are not harmful.)

Cholesterol is a type of blood lipid that is chemically more like a wax than a fat. It is produced naturally in the liver, and a small amount is necessary for the body to use as building blocks for sex hormones, cell membranes, and digestive secretions. However, by eating foods that contain high amounts of cholesterol and saturated fat, we build up excess cholesterol in our blood that can harden into plaque inside our arteries. So the lower the fat in your diet, the lower the cholesterol.

Many studies have corroborated Dr. Ornish's findings that reducing dietary fat will not just halt the progress of atherosclerotic plaques, it will actually improve the condition of the arteries. Blood pressure, and blood sugar too, was reduced in these studies—although high cholesterol doesn't cause high blood pressure or diabetes, it is probably a contributor since it adds to the total dysfunction of the cardiovascular system.

How Much Cholesterol Is Okay?

We have been told for years that if we keep our total cholesterol level below 200 mg/dl (milligrams per deciliter), we're okay. That is apparently no longer true for many individuals. Remember that some of us are more predisposed to heart disease than others. If you look at your risk factors (see chapter 2), you will have a pretty good barometer of where you stand and how much precaution you should take.

If you do have some risk factors or have already been diagnosed with heart disease, you should try to get your cholesterol down below 150 mg/dl. According to the long-term Framingham Heart Study, which has been going on for thirty-five years in Massachusetts, no one in the study who had cholesterol under 150 ever got a heart attack.

You should of course discuss your concern with your physician, particularly if he or she is satisfied with your levels hovering at 200. Some people—despite their best efforts— cannot bring their cholesterol levels down this low. You must also keep in mind that the ratio of your HDL to LDL is what your physician is really looking at, and if your HDL is over 65, you're in very good shape.

The New Secret to Combating Heart Disease: Soy Protein

A report in the *New England Journal of Medicine* from August 1995 stated that soy protein significantly lowers cholesterol in individuals whose cholesterol levels put them at high risk for heart disease. The higher the LDLs, the greater the benefit from eating soy products. A diet of 47 grams of soy protein daily (equivalent to about two soy burgers and an 8-ounce glass of soy milk) cuts cholesterol levels by approximately 9.3 percent in just one month, unless you have extremely high cholesterol to begin with. The studies found that individuals with levels over 300 benefited far more— their cholesterol was cut by 20 percent in a month.

Since a 10 to 15 percent reduction in blood cholesterol levels equals a 20 to 30 percent reduction in heart disease risk, just six months on a high soy diet—in combination, of course, with balanced nutrients, exercise, and smoking cessation—could change your entire cardiac picture. Another factor is that when you're consuming soy protein (tempeh or tofu or miso) as your main course, you have no room left for animal protein, which usually comes larded with fat.

Unlike most other methods of reducing cholesterol, where both the "bad" LDLs and the "good" HDLs are lowered, soy protein *only* reduces the LDLs and harmful triglycerides, leaving all the positive benefits of the plaque-fighting HDLs.

The helpful benefits to reduce heart disease risk kick in when you're eating at least 25 grams of soy daily (although twice that is recommended if your cholesterol levels are very high). A soy burger has about 18 grams of protein; a glass of soy milk has about 8, and a cake of tempeh or tofu has approximately 16 grams. You can also buy "No-Dogs" and fake sausages, available in most supermarkets; and you can drink soy milk and eat soy cheese and soy ice cream. An occasional bowl of miso soup when you're out at a Japanese restaurant will give you a little bit more protection.

Why Fiber Can Help Your Heart

We have been told for years to eat our roughage because it will keep us "regular," fight obesity, and help to protect us from colon cancer. The gastrointestinal claims of fiber are certainly important, but the cardiac benefits are what concern us the most here.

What Is Fiber and How Does It Affect the Heart?

Fiber is the indigestible cell-wall material of plants. Water-soluble fiber—found in oats and oat bran; fruits such as apples, blackberries, peaches, pears, plums; and dried peas and beans—can dissolve in water but not in your digestive tract.

The second type, water-insoluble fiber, survives intact in water or stomach acid.

Soluble fiber appears to enhance the cholesterol-lowering effect of a low-fat diet. When oat bran is added to such a diet, it can bring down LDLs by 24 percent and lower total cholesterol levels by 26 percent in just twenty-four weeks.

In one study a group was asked to increase their fiber intake by 6 grams daily. Over the twelve years of the study, after factoring in all other variables, it was shown that this increase brought a 25 percent reduction in deaths from coronary heart disease. People who switch to vegetarian diets (which obviously contain more fiber than omnivorous diets) are able to decrease mild or moderate hypertension.

People who eat high-fiber diets are less likely to develop diabetes (which is in itself a risk factor for heart disease), and switching to a high-fiber diet can help already established diabetics to improve blood sugar control, increase the body's sensitivity to insulin (which helps to use fats and sugars appropriately), lower cholesterol levels and blood pressure, and help in weight management (obesity is also a risk factor for heart disease).

How to Get More Fiber in Your Diet

If you eat an average American diet, you consume between 10 and 23 grams of fiber daily. But experts feel the optimum diet should contain between 25 and 35 grams. How do you know how much fiber you are eating? If you give up white bread for whole grain, consume your daily requirement of vegetables, always buy high-fiber cereals, and make sure you eat the skins on your potatoes and apples, you will be taking in at least 25 grams of fiber daily.

If you're making a casserole or meat loaf, sprinkle on some oat bran to thicken the mix. When you buy cereal, make sure it contains no less than 3 grams of fiber per serving. Instead of high-sugar, high-sodium cereals, switch to plain bran flakes or Uncle Sam's, which contains the high-fiber psyllium seed. Purchase or bake bread products using whole-grain flours. If you snack on chips and pretzels, switch to carrots, celery, and apples.

You may also wish to consider a natural-fiber supplement that comes as crackers or as a powder to be mixed with water or juice. Consult your physician as to the advisability of adding psyllium in this form to your diet.

Be sure to increase your consumption of this nutrient slowly, adding a few grams a week, so as not to upset your system. You could start with an extra apple or three prunes or one bowl of bran cereal. Drink lots of fluids to prevent bloating and gas, and don't overdo it. Taking in more than 35 grams of fiber a day may interfere with calcium absorption.

Some Help in Changing Your Eating Habits

The type of eating you've been doing all your life is so comfortable and familiar, it's difficult to consider anything else. However, the changes suggested here and the specific foods that will assist in your program will give you the most effective weapon in your arsenal of holistic care to combat heart disease.

The facts are very easy to absorb: The more fat and cholesterol you eat, the more plaque on your arteries, the more danger to your heart. The less fat and cholesterol, the less plaque. (There are individuals who are predisposed to create an excess of cholesterol, no matter their diet. However, most of us are able to adjust our LDLs and HDLs by modifying what we eat and how we move around.)

Keeping Good Food Around the House

If you don't buy junk food and always keep a larder full of nutritious food, you will always have what you need when you start to cook heart-healthy.

To cover all meals and impromptu healthy entertaining, you will need to stock some of the following staples:

BREAKFASTS

Whole grains (oats, millet, brown rice) to make muffins and breads

Oat groats, kasha

Cold whole-grain cereals (plain bran is best) with no sugar or salt

Skim milk or 1% milk

Flatbreads (Kavli crackers from Sweden)

Bagels

Egg whites

No-fat yogurt

Pure fruit spreads

Fresh fruits and juices

Low-fat Pam spray for muffin pans

Herbal teas

LUNCHES

Vegetables (starchy and nonstarchy)

Salad fixings

Corn tortillas (frozen) to which you can add lots of fillings

Variety of beans for homemade bean dip

Sardines in water

Water-packed tuna

Sparkling water

Limes and lemons

Fresh fruits and juices

Herbal teas

Hummus spread (dip made of chickpeas, tahini, garlic, lemon, and olive oil)

Soy products (tempeh, tofu, miso)

Soy milk
Air-popped popcorn

DINNERS
Vegetables (starchy and nonstarchy)
Whole grains
Stock or bouillon (you can make your own and freeze or buy salt-free canned stock)
Potatoes
Garlic and onions
Beans (pinto, navy, kidney, lentils, chickpeas—buy dried or reduced-sodium canned beans, then rinse before cooking)
Olive oil, canola oil
Vinegars of different varieties
Pasta of every variety
No-yolk noodles
Rice (long- and short-grain)
Canned whole tomatoes
Egg substitutes (read labels carefully to see oil content)
Spices and herbs
Garlic
Onions
Mustards
Salsa
Alfalfa and psyllium seeds (to be sprinkled into casseroles)
Wheat germ
Dried red chilis
Dried wild mushrooms
Fresh ginger

ONCE OR TWICE A WEEK (in 4-ounce portions ONLY)
Cold-seawater fish (cod, mackerel, salmon, sardines, herring)

Poultry without skin
Ground turkey
"Select" cuts of beef

Smart Cooking Tips to Help Your Heart

Once your larder is stocked and you've planned your menus, it's time to prepare your food in a way that will enhance the good qualities of low-fat eating.

Follow these tips for the different food groups:

BREAD, CEREAL, RICE, AND PASTA

- You can make your own breads by investing in a bread machine. This way you get to use the best ingredients for your heart, and you also know exactly what's in every loaf.
- If you do your own baking, always substitute 1% or 2% milk for whole milk or cream.
- Make your own granolas with different grains and raisins, but concentrate on oatmeal and bran as daily cereals.

VEGETABLE GROUP

- Vegetables can be baked, broiled, roasted, steamed, or poached. Don't boil them—water-soluble vitamins and minerals will vanish into the cooking water. You can eat them raw or juice them.
- Substitute lemon juice, soy sauce, chives, or salsa for butter and cheese on top of your vegetables.

FRUIT GROUP

- Eat uncooked fresh fruit, or toss with fruit juice or a dab of honey.

- When you have a craving for pie, make your own with a whole wheat crust and fresh fruit, with fruit juice instead of syrup to moisten it.

MILK, YOGURT, AND CHEESE GROUP

- In recipes that call for whole milk or cream, substitute skim milk thickened with cornstarch or evaporated skim milk.
- Substitute yogurt for sour cream.
- Substitute cottage cheese blended with skim milk for cream cheese. Flavor it with herbs and spices.

MEAT, POULTRY, FISH, AND LEGUMES

- You can bake, broil, roast, steam, poach, or boil.
- Before you cook meat, trim off all visible fat and discard.
- Before you cook poultry, take off the skin and discard.
- When cooking legumes, add flavorings to your cooking water. You can use bay leaves, onion, garlic, and whatever herb will complement your recipe.

EGGS

- If a recipe calls for egg yolks or whole eggs, use one yolk and make all the rest egg whites. You can color egg whites with turmeric. You can also use Egg Beaters or another egg substitute, as long as the oil content isn't too high.

FATS AND OILS

- You should not fry, sauté in fat, or dip foods in egg and batter before cooking them.
- You can occasionally use a small amount of monounsaturated fats—olive or canola oil—in your pan to flavor your vegetables, legumes, or meats.

- Use a nonstick vegetable shortening spray (olive oil is best) to coat the pan.
- You can "sauté" vegetables and meats in a wok, using a small amount of broth, wine, or tomato sauce to moisten them.
- Don't buy commercial salad dressings. Make your own with olive oil and vinegar or lemon juice.

FLAVORING
- Cut down on, or entirely cut out, salt in your food preparation and at the table if you have high blood pressure.
- Experiment with herbs such as dill, chives, parsley, taragon, curry, basil, and oregano in your cooking.
- There are also savory substitutes for salt (such as Mrs. Dash) that will add flavor to foods.
- You can use any of the following in preparation or at the table: lemon, mustard, ketchup, horseradish, salsa or taco sauce, vinegar, Worcestershire sauce.

Packaged, Prepared, and Restaurant Foods

If it comes in a package, or if it's served to you in a restaurant, you must be absolutely sure you know what you're eating. This isn't hard—all you have to do is learn to read a label and become comfortable with asking for what you want, cooked as you like it.

The FDA has now determined that all packaged food *must* include vital information that will tell us all we need to know about what we're going to put in our mouths. Most prepared foods list their ingredients in descending order of the amount contained in the food, and the label will tell you the percentage of fat calories. Stick with whole-grain, low-fat products, either homemade or store-bought.

When you're in a restaurant, you're the boss. First look for little hearts in the margin of the menu to see whether the establishment you're in serves "heart-healthy" meals.

If not, you can select pasta or a vegetarian plate; you can have a nice piece of fish or poultry without skin. Be very particular about asking for the details of the sauces.

Make sure you ask for

- baked, broiled, roasted, or steamed only
- salad dressing on the side
- vegetables cooked without butter
- pasta or rice with tomato-based, not cream-based, sauces
- salsa instead of hollandaise, béarnaise, or any egg-yolk-based sauce
- an egg-white omelet
- fresh fruit cup in its natural juices or lightly sugared

Enjoy Your Meals

When you've put so much loving care into shopping and preparing what you eat, take the time to eat it right. Think about the wonderful aromas and flavors; think about how good you will feel on a diet that contains only elements that are beneficial to your heart.

Savor each meal and eat when you're hungry, stopping when you're satisfied. Don't eat standing up or in front of the TV. Make sure you chew carefully, tasting each morsel, relishing the idea of doing preventive cardiac care in your own kitchen.

Exercise—The Greatest Boon to the Heart

We were meant to get up and move. Before there were cars, buses, trains, and planes, humans spent most of their time being active and were far less prone to diseases of affluence such as cancer and heart disease.

It has been amply proved that exercise reduces your risk of heart disease, stroke, hypertension, diabetes, and obesity.

That means fewer heart attacks and bypasses. And a far healthier, more comfortable life.

Exercise

- lowers LDLs and raises HDLs
- lowers systolic and diastolic blood pressures
- lowers triglycerides
- decreases the stickiness of blood platelets, making it harder for clots to build up and block arteries
- thins the blood so that it can move through blood vessels more easily
- strengthens the heart muscle, along with all the other muscles in the body
- keeps you motivated to eat well so that you can usually lose weight if you have to and maintain it if you're already in an optimum weight range
- alleviates tension and elevates your mood so that you actually want to stick with your preventive care program, because it increases your production of beta-endorphins, those neurotransmitters in the brain that give a feeling of well-being.

There has been some controversy about how much exercise really makes a difference. We know that *getting no exercise at all is extremely dangerous* to our health—it's been calculated that being sedentary multiplies your risk of heart attack by a factor of 1.9, which means that 205,000 heart attack deaths a year could be prevented simply by adding aerobic activity to our daily regimen.

But how much activity is enough? Although the most recent data say that you have to be working hard (five or six days a week, half an hour a day) at vigorous aerobic exercise in order to live appreciably longer, most studies agree that *moderate daily activity,* such as walking or biking, is enough to prevent heart attacks and keep the cardiovascular system fit. One study divided subjects into five categories (from most fit to least fit) and found that the death rate was highest in the least fit but declined greatly in the next category up. The second level of exercisers did really well. In this group men had death rates that were 60 percent lower and women 48 percent lower than those who did nothing at all. The more effort you put out, evidently, the better off you are.

What Will Exercise Do for You If You Have Heart Disease?

Suppose you've already had a heart attack or undergone bypass surgery? What kind of benefit do you get from exercise in a rehabilitation program? In a meta-analysis (a grouping of many different studies) of four thousand individuals who stuck with their cardiac rehab programs, there was a 25 percent reduction in the rate of a second attack and overall death rate. Aerobic activity, the type that raises your heart rate to its maximum safe level, is a way of increasing your capacity to exercise without angina or shortness of breath.

As you become more fit, you can open up atherosclerotic blockages throughout your body—individuals who found walking uncomfortable before starting a program often find that their peripheral blood flow is so much better after a few months, they take up hiking. A renewed or less problematic sexual life can be an additional bonus of a good exercise program. Men who've had sexual difficulty find that they can achieve and maintain an erection because of increased blood flow to the genitals, and women tend to be more orgasmic for the same reason.

Aerobic Exercise Plus Isometric

You'll have a stronger heart after you've been working out for three months, but that's not your major goal. In order to have your heart respond well to exercise, the rest of your body and mind must get with the plan as well. This means you have to combine all the elements of fitness into your daily schedule. You need the following:

- *Aerobic activity,* which pumps your heart rate to 70 percent of its maximum rate. This is the type of movement that gets you sweating (which also releases toxins from your body) and increases your respiration.
- *Flexibility exercises,* which will ensure that the tendons and ligaments around the bone are getting a good workout. One of the chief reasons that people drop out of exercise programs is injury—but if you warm up properly before starting to jog, hike, dance, do martial arts, or even walk or swim, you'll avoid hurting yourself.
- *Strength exercises.* To make sure that your whole body is in shape and can withstand the burden of increased stress on the bones and joints, weight training is a real boon. This type of activity is called *isometric,* or static, exercise. Although blood pressure increases as your heart works harder to lift, you're not going to be doing such hard work that it constricts your blood vessels. You will instead be lifting light free weights or using low-resistance weights on a Nautilus machine and doing more repetitions. Even eighty- and ninety-year-olds in nursing homes have benefited from increasing upper-body strength by lifting two- or three-pound weights in each hand—many are able to throw away their canes and walkers after a monitored program of weight training.
- *Endurance exercises.* You're not aiming for a quick burst of energy to take you across a finish line. You are rather hoping to be able to move easily in space over time at increasingly difficult levels of activity. By working on endurance (tai chi and yoga are particularly good for this—see chapter 4), you will build long-range go-power.

Adding Exercise to Your Life

Set goals for yourself, and give yourself rewards for reaching them. Don't be upset if you fall behind, and by no means count yourself a failure if you do less than you anticipated. If you're doing *something,* you're helping your heart.

You must start slowly and work your way into activities that will stress your heart at an increasing rate. This way you'll avoid injury and the anxious feeling that the program you've selected is too difficult. It is much more important to do some moderate exercise every day than to overtrain several times a week. If you are a very healthy person when you start your exercise schedule, you will be attempting to raise your heart rate to a maximum rate calculated by this formula:

---

220 − your age × 70 percent
(For example, if you are fifty years old, it would be
220 − 50 = 170 × 70 percent = 119 beats per minute.)

If you are recuperating from a heart attack or have already been diagnosed with heart disease, 70 percent may be too high. Your physician must prescribe the correct percentage for your ability.

In order to know how hard you're working, you have to learn to take your own pulse. Count the number of heartbeats by feeling the pulse in your neck or wrist for 15 seconds, then multiply by 4. Take your pulse before you start, then, after you've been exercising for about 20 minutes, then again as you recover. As you get into better shape, you'll find that your heart rate gets back to its normal resting rhythm more quickly.

You are aiming for an aerobic fitness level that will improve the pumping action of the heart muscle. When you exercise, your muscles demand more oxygen. Naturally they get this oxygen as it is carried in the blood. As you inhale deeply during strenuous exercise, your heart beats faster and contracts more powerfully. Over time your heart accommodates to the new demands put on it and is able to recover more quickly when you relax after exercising. This means that the heart—and the arteries and veins that supply it with blood—becomes more efficient as you work out more.

How to Stick with an Exercise Program

Luckily, exercise is addictive for most people. Although addiction is not a word that's usually associated with health, the truth of the matter is that there is a quality of wanting and needing more when you're feeling so good and doing so well. Exercise relaxes you, and as you feel more relaxed, you crave that feeling all the time.

Which is fine, because to keep your heart in good shape, you have to be in this for the long run. Starting a program today is like the first day you begin piano lessons. You can play the scales, even a few easy melodies, but it will take concentrated practice time to master a Beethoven piano concerto. Similarly, it takes months to build up stamina and expertise in whatever exercise mode you choose—but by doing so you build in more healthy years on your life span.

If you have already had a heart attack, exercise can help to prevent a second one. Those patients who participate in a cardiac rehabilitation program have more motivation to get well faster and may possibly improve the length as well as the quality of their lives.

Always consult your health care practitioner about what and how much you can do. You might also want to sit down with a friend or family member and plot out a program you can do together. Then get yourself a good pair of walking or cross-training shoes. Progress a little every week, every month, every year. If you move your body every single day of your life, you may not only avoid a heart attack but also reduce numerous risk factors for heart disease.

Overcoming Exercise Reluctance

Although exercise can be addictive, it's not always easy to get hooked. There are actually very few individuals (even professional athletes) who always love their daily practice. It is grueling, boring, and you occasionally reach plateaus or feel as if you are slipping backward.

The philosophy of all holistic health practice is moderation in everything. That means not knocking yourself out in the interests of getting ahead in your chosen sport faster and getting your heart into even better shape. You don't want to contribute to the depressing statistic that only half of those who start an exercise program stick with it. Whether you're beginning a preventive-care regimen and really want to re-vamp your life or your physician has enrolled you in a cardiac rehabilitation plan, there is no legitimate excuse to quit once you've started!

TIPS TO HELP YOU KEEP EXERCISING DAILY:

- Get social support and/or an exercise partner. A study presented at the Society for Behavioral Medicine showed that 92 percent of those who had a partner who agreed to exercise with them kept going: 50 percent of the single people quit within the year. If someone is depending on you to hit a ball back over the net or walk that country mile, you know you can't drop out.
- Be flexible. If you can't walk outside because it's below zero, go to a mall and cover some ground. If you have an early-morning appointment and will have to miss your regular tennis game, arrange with your partner to get a court for that evening. If you're rigid about how and when you exercise, and you have to skip a few days

because of a cold or an unmanageable schedule, you may feel you've failed and never go back. But if you stay loose, you'll realize you can get back on track easily.

- Set realistic goals. Don't think about running a marathon or bench-pressing your own weight. If you plot yourself a short-term goal, you'll find a little success. When you've accomplished one goal, plan the next, and challenge yourself a little more. Eventually you'll be quite an expert at what you do and be able to teach others.
- Don't expect that exercise will help you lose weight. It may, but since muscle weighs more than fat, you may see no changes on the scale at all unless you were significantly overweight to start with.
- Listen to your body. If you're feeling pain, weakness, difficulty breathing, or anything that is not normal for you, stop at once, sit down, and breathe. Make sure you inform your physician about any and all symptoms when you are physically active.
- In order to develop a healthy addiction to exercising, think about it when you're not doing it. Visualization *plus* practice has been found to help athletes to improve their technique. So if you can see yourself swimming the entire width of the lake beside your summer cabin, you may just be able to accomplish it.

Tips to Add More Activity to Your Busy Day

In addition to an organized exercise schedule, there are many other ways to stay active without taking any extra time from your day:

- Walk or bike to your destination instead of driving.
- Walk down the hall to a colleague's office instead of calling or E-mailing.
- Park several blocks away from your destination and walk the rest of the way.

- When you take your children or grandchildren to the park, play with them instead of sitting on a bench and watching.
- Take the stairs instead of the elevator or escalator.
- If you're watching TV, get up to change channels instead of using the remote control.
- Put a piece of exercise equipment—a treadmill, rowing machine, StairMaster, or exercise bike—in front of your TV and always use it when you watch a program.

Exercise will do more than prevent a heart attack. It will make you feel better, stronger, more relaxed, and will give you an indefinable "glow." And when people start telling you how well you look and asking for your secret, don't keep it to yourself. They need to exercise just as much as you do!

Lifestyle: How to Adopt Good Habits and Curtail Bad Ones

Habits are easy to make and very difficult so break, so we might as well make ones that will improve our health. Smoking cigarettes, drinking caffeine and alcohol, using recreational drugs, and sleeping too little can seriously damage the body and mind and make heart disease a real possibility.

Which habits do you have? What can you eliminate immediately and what's going to take you some time? You do need willpower and a lot of social support—perhaps even a professional therapeutic program—to overcome the effects of their influence. Look at the following list and order it in terms of your own priorities:

Smoking

Cigarette smoking accounts for 200,000 cardiac deaths a year, and the risk of a heart attack in a smoker is twice that of a nonsmoker. Just one cigarette narrows coronary arteries by 35 percent, and this effect stays in the heart for at least half an hour. If you smoke a pack a day, you are reducing the ability of your blood to carry oxygen (since it's so full of carbon monoxide) and putting yourself at risk for angina, arrhythmias, and possibly a heart attack. Smoking contributes to blood clots and to constricted blood vessels in the legs, kidneys, heart, and brain. The Center for Disease Control estimates that every cigarette you smoke lowers your life expectancy by seven minutes. Living with a smoker and inhaling passively raises your risk of death by 30 percent.

No, it's not easy to stop, but just one year after quitting, your risk of heart disease is cut in half; fifteen years after, your risk is exactly that of a never-smoker. If you are a smoker of cigarettes, cigars, pipes, or a chewer of tobacco, you are being kept in thrall to your habit by the addictive nature of nicotine, which incidentally also raises blood pressure. A program (sometimes accompanied by use of a patch or Nicorette gum), is the most effective way for most people to stop smoking. Hypnosis is often helpful, but generally only if you are taught to hypnotize yourself.

Here are some more tips to help you quit:

- Chew sugarless gum, have a glass of water, or eat a carrot stick when you get the urge for a cigarette.
- If you tend to light up when you drink a cup of coffee, switch to tea or flavored sparkling water. If you always smoke when you're on the telephone, make sure you have a pencil and pad to play with as you talk.
- Avoid friends who smoke while you're trying to quit—or ask them not to smoke when you're around.
- Join a support group. This can be one of the most useful tools for maintaining a new and difficult pattern of self-care.

Alcohol and Recreational Drugs

The good news is that a little alcohol (one 6-ounce glass of wine or 12 ounces of beer daily) is good for your heart because it bumps up HDL levels. In six weeks a daily glass of wine boosts your HDLs by 5 to 10 points—which equals a 40 percent reduction in cardiac risk. It may also reduce blood clotting by acting on platelets and fibrinogen levels, and it may assist in balancing blood sugar. But just a little more than the minimum allowance can be extremely bad for your heart—it may contribute to hypertension, arrhythmias, strokes, and brain hemorrhages. It may trigger angina attacks and damage the heart muscle, which can lead to congestive heart failure.

If you're trying to cut down, don't spend time with friends who drink or use drugs.

All recreational drugs are dangerous to your general well-being and can be lethal for your heart. Amyl nitrate (poppers) is a particularly deadly pharmaceutical product, and marijuana, cocaine, and heroin are not just addictive, they can do actual damage to the blood vessels and to your ability to move oxygen in the blood.

Caffeine

Coffee and other caffeineated products (tea, chocolate, cocoa, and soda) appear to raise total cholesterol levels; however, experts are not sure exactly how coffee consumption affects the prognosis of heart disease. (Part of the problem is that individuals who drink coffee often smoke and eat high-fat diets.) High doses of caffeine also create irregular heartbeats—along with the "jitters"—in many individuals. Cardiac problems are exacerbated in caffeine-drinking smokers, particularly if they have high blood pressure.

Caffeine is a nervous system stimulant. The addictive nature of this stimulant is caused by its ability to impart a jolt of energy to the body. What really happens when you drink a cup of coffee is similar to the "fight or flight" response you get when you're anxious or tense—the brain responds and tells the adrenal glands to pour out the stress hormones adrenaline and noradrenaline. It will take from three days to two weeks to break the habit and establish a new natural sense of alertness.

Sleep

Sleep affords the body a chance to rest and recuperate, and helps to strengthen the immune system. It also imparts the energy necessary to respond to difficult physical and emotional situations when we're awake. Make sure you are tired when you go to bed (moderate daily exercise will ensure that you get a good night's rest), and don't nap during the day. A natural sleeping remedy is a cup of warm milk whirred up in a blender with a banana (both contain tryptophan, an amino acid that promotes sleep). If you typically go to bed late, try retiring fifteen minutes earlier each night, and set the alarm clock for a specific time in the morning.

The Golden Rules Can Save Your Life

Diet, exercise, and lifestyle change are for everyone, whether you have already been diagnosed with heart disease or not. And these are principles we can pass on to the next generation as well. If in childhood and adolescence we start eating, moving, and living right, we won't have to make drastic changes as we approach the age where a heart attack might be imminent.

There are other ways, of course, to maintain terrific cardiac health. In the next chapter we'll show you how to use your mind and spirit to manage stress and enhance the results of sticking to your three golden rules.

LIFE INSURANCE WEIGHT TABLES (LBS.)

WOMEN

Height	Small Frame	Medium Frame	Midpoint Reference	+10%	+20%	Large Frame
4'10"	102–111	109–121	115	127	138	118–131
4'11"	103–113	111–123	117	129	140	120–134
5' 0"	104–115	113–126	120	132	144	122–137
5' 1"	106–118	115–129	122	134	146	125–140
5' 2"	108–121	118–132	125	138	150	128–143
5' 3"	111–124	121–135	128	141	154	131–147
5' 4"	114–127	124–138	131	144	157	134–151
5' 5"	117–130	127–141	134	147	161	137–155
5' 6"	120–133	130–144	137	151	164	140–159
5' 7"	123–136	133–147	140	154	168	143–163
5' 8"	126–139	136–150	143	158	172	146–167
5' 9"	129–142	139–153	146	161	175	149–170
5'10"	132–145	142–156	149	164	179	152–173
5'11"	135–148	145–159	152	167	182	155–176
6' 0"	138–151	148–162	155	170	186	158–179

LIFE INSURANCE WEIGHT TABLES (LBS.)

MEN

Height	Small Frame	Medium Frame	Midpoint Reference	+10%	+20%	Large Frame
5' 2"	128–134	131–141	136	150	163	138–150
5' 3"	130–136	133–143	138	152	166	140–153
5' 4"	132–138	135–145	140	154	168	142–156
5' 5"	134–140	137–148	142	156	170	144–160
5' 6"	136–142	139–151	145	160	174	146–164
5' 7"	138–145	142–154	148	163	178	149–168
5' 8"	140–148	145–157	151	166	181	152–172
5' 9"	142–151	148–160	154	169	185	155–176
5'10"	144–154	151–163	157	173	188	158–180
5'11"	146–157	154–166	160	172	192	161–184
6' 0"	149–160	157–170	163	179	196	164–188
6' 1"	152–164	160–174	167	184	200	168–192
6' 2"	155–168	164–178	171	188	205	172–197
6' 3"	158–172	167–185	174	191	209	176–202
6' 4"	162–176	171–187	179	197	215	181–207

CHAPTER FOUR

Stress Management and the Mind-Body Therapies

We are well aware that heart disease produces physical symptoms—we can see the condition of blocked arteries and faulty valves on diagnostic tests and read cholesterol and blood levels that tell us something is physiologically wrong.

But what is less apparent is that heart disease also has emotional and mental components, which can be dealt with effectively. At the same time that you are modifying your diet, exercising, and improving your lifestyle, you can also be learning to control physical symptoms with mental and emotional resources.

In this chapter we will talk about stress and its opposite, relaxation. Then we'll outline four mind-body techniques: yoga, tai chi chuan, visualization, and meditation, which have all been used successfully in cardiac prevention and rehabilitation programs.

The Nature of Stress and Heart Disease

There are many mechanisms that disturb the heart function, and one of them is the powerful effect of stress on our mind and body. When the mind perceives an event as stressful, we experience a pounding heart, clammy hands, grinding in the stomach, and tense muscles. As soon as the brain registers fear or distress, it starts a chain of biochemical messages coursing through the blood and nervous system in a response known as ''fight or flight.''

Every system—the cardiovascular, musculoskeletal, endocrine, nervous, and immune systems—all react to internal stress events over which we feel we have no control. As our brain tells the body that something bad is occurring, a chain of chemical reactions begins. The adrenal glands, part of the endocrine system, pick up the warning signal and produce three hormones—*adrenaline, noradrenaline,* and *cortisol.* These substances wreak havoc on our cells, helping to start a reaction that raises blood pressure and heartbeat, keeps LDL cholesterol high, and even blocks immune responses.

If this persists, day after day, we reach a state of chronic hyperarousal. Our stress level no longer goes up and down with given events, but instead stays raised, so that we produce these ''struggle'' hormones all the time. The various physiological reactions caused by our emotional response never get a chance to dissipate—pressure stays elevated, arrhythmias persist, LDLs circulate abundantly in the blood—all of which can do damage to the delicate interior of blood vessel walls.

In the meantime we find that we can't sleep well (and thus rest the mind and body so that we can handle another day's stresses), and develop headaches, backaches, and other unpleasant symptoms. We may compensate by adopting negative coping behaviors—abusing alcohol and tobacco, overeating, and abandoning our daily exercise schedule.

Although the body reacts quickly to adapt to stress, there is a point beyond which it can't take any more. Over years, due to the accumulation of stressors such as a bad marriage, an unfulfilling job, the death of a parent, a child in trouble, as well as the daily annoyances such as car breakdowns and the nasty comments of strangers or colleagues, the systems that have protected us start to break down. Dr. Hans Selye, the father of modern stress management, describes the *diseases of adaptation* as the way the body copes over time. The loss of motivation and depression of a generally stressful life may lead to heart attacks, cancers, and other chronic conditions.

Some individuals have a higher reacting mechanism than others—the people we label type A seem to want to take a bite out of life. Their counterparts, the type Bs, who are laid-back and low pressure, usually fend off disease the way they do everything else—by ignoring it.

The interesting thing about type As, who were first studied as those at higher risk for heart disease, is that they often cope well with stress. They regard each difficult moment as a challenge, or *eu*-stress (''good'' stress) instead of a terrible failing, or *dis*-stress (''bad'' stress). These people thrive on the excitement of looking at a bad situation, wrestling with it, and dealing with it effectively. Because type As tend to see stress as an immediate issue that can be handled, they are usually not in terrible jeopardy of doing damage to their heart.

Those who can't see an end to the stress, however, are those in the most danger. Prolonged, protracted, unalleviated stress is the kind that raises LDL cholesterol as it pumps in the stress hormones that may cause negative changes in the blood vessels. Those who take on too many burdens and seem to feel that they can never do enough or please enough people have been designated as type E (having to be everything to everybody) by psychologist Harriet Braiker.

The longing to be perfect, and despair at the fact that this is an impossible goal, has sent many people to the emergency room with a heart attack. What happens is that the fight-or-flight response never gets closure—the tightened muscles, the knot in the stomach, the arteries that constrict in order to "hold on to" the blood should danger arise—just don't go away. And when arteries narrow, blood clots can form, spasms can occur, and heart attacks can happen.

The Trick of Managing Your Stress: Staying in the Moment

Part of the emotional burden of stress is that most of us are always looking back into the past and forward into the future without giving due consideration to the present moment. As soon as you learn *not* to anticipate and to deal only with what's on your plate at any particular point in time, you will be able to manage your stress far more efficiently.

If you can stop the fight-or-flight response, or just control it, you may be able to reduce your cardiac risk. Dr. Dean Ornish, head of the Preventive Medicine Research Institute in California, has helped those with chronic heart disease reverse their condition, partly by using the power of the mind. Dr. Jon Kabat-Zinn, at the University of Massachusetts Medical Center, has found that meditation and hatha yoga are part of a comprehensive treatment that can help prevent heart attacks and strengthen the life force of participants. Dr. Martin Milner, of the Center for Natural Therapy in Portland, Oregon, uses these techniques as part of a well-rounded program of cardiac preventive and restorative care.

How can you stay calm when all those around you are losing their heads?

You need a technique that will allow you to *relax*. Unfortunately in this day, when stress is such a present part of our lives, when most of us experience anger and tension on a daily, sometimes hourly basis, we have to be taught to think less, to focus more, to abandon expectations and mostly to *let go*.

Techniques to Manage Stress

The most important elements in a good stress management program are the following:

- Participation in a daily structured type of mental calming, such as meditation, prayer, yoga, or tai chi chuan.
- Time management, to learn where your priorities lie and how best to organize what you have to do—and what you want to do. Even if you feel that all your stresses have to be taken care of immediately, you can actually only deal with one at a time.
- Behavior modification—to show how you can control even the smallest reactions to stress, such as nail biting, junk-food consumption, and poor sleep habits, as well as the big ones, such as smoking and alcohol abuse. Make yourself a chart of when you do a certain behavior and mark it faithfully. Give yourself incentives to change the behavior, as well as a reward at the end.
- Goal setting—to learn what you really want out of life. Write down five weekly, monthly, and yearly goals, and make yourself a long-range goal as well. (This is not contradictory to living in the present moment! Goal setting is a way of grounding yourself and selecting a path on which all your present moments will follow logically.)
- Creating a support system so that you always have someone to call or visit when you feel overwhelmed. If you learn to delegate responsibility, both at work and at home, you can take some pressure off yourself. No, the jobs will not be done exactly as you would do them. But you will grow to appreciate others' competence as you learn to lower your standards for perfection.

Stress Quiz

You probably realize that you have stress in your life—but do you know how much you're dealing with? The following quiz will help you assess your stress problem:

1. Is it always necessary for you to get control of people and situations?
2. Are you a leader?
3. Do you find it difficult to take criticism or follow directions?
4. Do you feel that your work is never done?
5. Does every tiny detail bother you if it isn't done to your satisfaction?
6. Do you make everyone else's problems your own?
7. Do you never take time for yourself?
8. Do you take on more tasks than it's possible for you to accomplish?
9. Do you rush from one activity to the next without allowing any time in between?
10. Do you eat, walk, talk quickly?
11. Do you finish other people's sentences for them?
12. Do you find it difficult to keep quiet and listen to others?
13. Does it take you a long time to fall asleep at night?
14. Do you get unreasonably angry at other drivers on the road?
15. Is it hard for you to wait on line?
16. Do you put off responsibilities until the last minute, then race to meet a deadline?
17. Are you impatient with others, particularly if they're slow or deliberate?
18. Do other people often disappoint you?
19. Do you try to make decisions for your partner or children instead of allowing them to decide what they want to do?

20. Do you feel it necessary to "fix" things immediately in your relationships or work situations instead of letting them come to their natural conclusion over time?

If the number of times you answered yes is 15 or more, you are under a great deal of stress and should begin some stress reduction program or technique. If your score is 10 or less, you're in pretty good shape. But regardless of your score, you should make a concerted effort to structure some quiet time—prayer, meditation, yoga, or tai chi—into your week.

The Mind-Body Techniques

One of the reasons that the body reacts to stress by developing symptoms that may eventually turn into a serious cardiac condition is that the mind and body are not communicating properly. The missed signals that would strengthen the immune system and allow the decrease in neurotransmitter flow create energetic blockages that may lead to "shear stresses" in the blood vessels that can damage the arteries over time.

The goal of mind-body therapies such as meditation, yoga, and tai chi chuan is to bring the mind and body back into a harmonious alignment. All of these disciplines teach the practitioner slowly and painstakingly to concentrate, focus, and use the energy within the body for practical benefits.

All of the bodywork aims to stimulate the nervous and lymphatic systems, to stretch and relax muscles, and to improve circulation. More important, these healing types of movement work internally, allowing you to clear your mind and relax, letting go of all the various stresses that may be contributing to your heart condition.

Breathing Is the Key to Mind-Body Therapies

Take a deep breath. Don't hold it, but let it course through your system. Let it out slowly and evenly. Do you notice the peace that's just settled into your body? You are suddenly relaxed, and even the most annoying or difficult problems you've got seem more workable.

Most of us take breathing for granted, but we must really make a study of this instinctive behavior if we want to have healthy hearts. Breathing affords better oxygenation to all tissues and at the same time removes excess carbon dioxide—our major toxic gas—from the body. It also allows us to relax tense muscles and shift emotional gears.

Oxygen is the fuel that keeps the heart going. It revitalizes this core mechanism that serves as the central feeding system for all the organs of the body. If we don't breathe, our heart doesn't pump, and consequently we don't see or hear, think or feel.

Sometimes people are afraid to breathe properly because they're nervous about taking in *too* much oxygen and hyperventilating. This abnormal pattern of heightened breathing makes you feel like you can't get enough air. But this can't happen when you learn to control the breath, even when you're anxious. When you hyperventilate, what's actually happening is that you're not getting enough oxygen and are getting rid of too much CO_2, which makes you light-headed. If you let this pattern run amok, you can black out—which will allow your body to relax and your breathing to return to normal.

In order to do any of the mind-body therapies, from yoga and tai chi to the more esoteric Feldenkrais, Alexander technique, bioenergetics, or Trager, you have to be able to focus your breath and consciously let it help you to relax.

How to Breathe

You knew how to breathe when you were a baby but have since lost the knack. However, regaining this ability isn't difficult and can be quickly mastered.

Babies breathe from their bellies. They allow the intake of air to propel oxygen from their bellies upward to their lungs. As they exhale, the outrush of air flattens the stomach area.

Adults breathe from their upper chest and shoulders. If you think of that moment in your doctor's office when a stethoscope comes near your heart, you'll recognize your instinctive reaction of pushing your chest in and out so that your doctor can get a reading on your heart rate.

But in doing so, only a shallow breath and the least amount of oxygen is allowed to enter the body. You don't have to concentrate on the lungs—they will expand anyway each time you inhale. Just forget about inflating the chest, and instead let the inspiration move from belly to back and kidneys up the spinal column to your head.

To get your breathing working for you, lie on your back on the floor or on a hard surface. Initially as you concentrate on your breath, you will probably notice your torso moving up and down. Now place your hand on your belly, about three inches below your waistband, and press down to force air into this region. Now relax your hand and see how your belly "bounces back." Watch the easy action of your hand moving up and down as you breathe in and out. Try to keep any effort out of your chest—pretend that all of your body is concentrated on that one point below your waist.

Practice this exercise five times the first day, eight the next, and ten thereafter until you are getting a substantial breath that feels comfortable and relaxed.

Next stand up in front of a mirror and blow into a balloon, using only your belly to do the inflating and deflating. Try not to use any breath from your chest at all and again watch the action of your stomach as the air moves in and out of you.

When you feel that this type of belly breathing is natural for you, sit in a hard-backed chair, or cross-legged on the floor, and simply pay attention to your breath. Clear your mind of other thoughts and concerns and just see the clear stream of air entering and leaving you, as though it were a flag wafting in the breeze.

If you experience shortness of breath, a feeling that you can't get enough air, or heart palpitations, stop immediately and return to normal breathing. Very often beginners try too much too quickly. Let several hours pass before you practice again, and reduce the number of breaths and depth of the breath you're taking.

Breathing can be done in conjunction with visualization. As you inhale, think of moving the breath from your center to your various organs. If you happen to have a particular symptom, an ache, or a pain, you can funnel energy to it by moving the breath to that particular area and concentrating on healing. You can also send the breath to your heart, or move it up your spine and down your head and torso to your center in order to balance body, mind, and spirit.

Visualization or Guided Imagery

Certain proven relaxation techniques that involve imagining a scene and putting yourself inside it have been shown to relieve stress and actually alter what used to be thought of as involuntary physiological responses. How does this phenomenon occur?

The brain, seat of the imagination, controls all of the major functions of the body via the hypothalamus and the pituitary, the glands that signal other glands to produce hormones to regulate sleep, blood chemistry, metabolism, temperature, immune system performance, and many other essential functions. The brain is also linked by the vagus nerve to the thymus gland just above the heart cavity. The thymus, one of the lymph glands in the immune system, produces white blood cells that fight disease. So as the brain directs healing energy through the nerves to this gland, we have an increase in beneficial T-cell production.

As you are healing your body by linking it more securely to brain mechanisms, you are also learning to change your own adaptation to pressure and stress. Visualization allows you to focus and problem-solve without the added distraction of hundreds of other thoughts. It lets you reach goals you may not even believe you can achieve, giving you control where you thought you had none.

Visualization allows you to become more positive-thinking, creatively dispelling fears and working from the perspective of a more confident attitude. It allows you to go inside yourself and reflect on who you are and how you came to this place. And finally, it lets you relax as you take care of the discomfort or symptom at hand.

This specific healing technique asks the practitioner to imagine her illness in terms of a concrete object and change it in her mind. If you have a valve malfunction, for example, you might think of the leaflets of that valve as swinging doors, opening and shutting in a regular rhythm. You may want to suggest to a narrowed artery that it is opening and expanding like a garden hose with water coursing through it. If you have coronary blockages, you might imagine a tiny drill, working its way through the fatty deposits in your arteries, gently clearing the path. With this technique you empower yourself to relieve the source of illness mentally. Studies have shown that cancer patients who used guided imagery in addition to their chemotherapy were able to reduce the size of their tumors over a six-month period more effectively than those who used no imagery and only chemotherapy.

Use the sample visualization that follows or create your own. There are just a few easy guidelines to keep in mind:

- Give yourself ample time—at least twenty minutes—for each visualization.
- Create a calm, quiet environment for yourself. It's best to do your visualization in a space with good ventilation and dim lighting.
- Breathe calmly and slowly throughout the exercise, no matter what the subject matter.
- At the end of the visualization allow yourself to come back slowly to real time. Let your eyes relax open.

Sample Visualization: An Open Heart

Empty your mind of thought and concentrate on your breath. Allow it to enter your body easily, like a gently flowing stream of water. When you are ready to exhale, see the breath moving out of you, leaving a core of energy behind.

Now take the breath deeper into your body, and feel it mix with your blood. Like an alchemist, you can prepare this mixture so that it touches every part of your body as it runs its internal course. See the oxygen stir your blood, washing the bad cholesterol off your arteries, reinforcing the presence of the good cholesterol. Imagine the power this red blood of life gives to your heart itself.

Now see the heart muscle, moving rhythmically inside you, like a racehorse hitting its stride. You have the power to keep that beat steady and strong, revitalizing you and calming your mind. You have no anxieties, no fears; your heart can bring its healing properties to any cell that needs help. Imagine the heart and the blood that feeds it as your staunchest allies, supporting you through your days and nights. See within yourself the intricate network of blood vessels, flexible and elastic as rubber bands, stretching as they need to to accommodate your blood pressure and flow.

Look directly at the heart. Watch it expand and contract, and then push aside your traditional image of a human heart. Open up your heart, push back its borders until just its outline is visible. In the center, now, is a pulsing light that gives beauty and constancy to the whole structure.

Come back to the calming breath that has taken you on this journey. Let your lungs and belly open and close, nurturing your body and mind with energy. Slowly allow your eyes to relax open.

Meditation

Similar to prayer, the various types of meditation are comforting methods of quieting the mind. The goal of meditating is not to remove all stimulation but rather to concentrate on one sound, one word, one image, or one's breath for a protracted period of time. Herbert Benson, M.D., a professor at Harvard Medical School, who coined the phrase *the relaxation response,* found that blood pressure was lowered, heart rate slowed, and muscle tension decreased during meditation. He documented the fact that oxygen needs of the body are lessened during meditation and that arrhythmias are not as frequent.

The particular types of meditation (Buddhist; Taoist; or TM, Transcendental Meditation) all have their own approaches. However, they all have the same goal in mind, which is to create peace of mind that will heal the body.

How to Meditate

Meditation is usually practiced as you sit cross-legged on a cushion on the floor, but you can sit in a chair, stand up, or walk and meditate.

Sitting meditation is not easy, particularly at first, when mind and body try to rebel against an unnatural position and the attempt to "do nothing." Your back may get tired and your feet or legs will probably fall asleep.

Don't alleviate the discomfort. Instead shift your concentration away from the pain to your breath. Let it calm you and assure you that nothing is wrong. Start to relax one body part after the next, using the breath to teach tense joints and muscles how to let go. The more you practice, the less pain you will feel and the more you'll be able to use breathing as a tool to help you.

It's not necessary to make the mind a complete void—as a matter of fact, trying to clear every thought away is futile for most Americans, who aren't accustomed to "nonthinking." Instead of erasing thought, allow thoughts to pass through similar to watching scenery from a train window. As soon as you have linked on to one image, let it go. As the next one comes to you, see it or feel it, and let it go. The more you sit quietly and give yourself the chance to focus your breathing and energy, the sooner you will be able to relinquish control of mental imagery.

One type of meditation often recommended for beginners is using the breath as your sole focus. Direct all of your attention to the inhalation and exhalation and keep the rhythm of your breathing as even as possible. You may also meditate on a single word, such as *Heart* or *Love* or even a sound such as *Om*.

Another type of meditation, known as mindfulness meditation, where you focus your attention on the one thing you are currently doing, is also useful for novices as well as advanced meditators. You can do anything at all mindfully— Jon Kabat-Zinn, who has popularized this technique, suggests eating a raisin. You hold it, feel its texture, think about its history as a grape, smell it, roll it around on your lip, place it between your lips and then remove it, lick it and experience the brief sweetness, and finally place it in your mouth. You then concentrate on the flow of saliva as you think about hunger, eating, and whether you like the taste of raisins. You pass the raisin around your mouth and see how your taste buds react. Chew slowly, thirty times, releasing the full flavor into your mouth. Postpone swallowing as long as possible as you consider the physical process of ingesting this particular raisin. At last you swallow, being aware of the remnants of raisin in your teeth, the lingering flavor on your tongue.

How can this exercise teach your heart to relax and work better? If you are able to use each moment profitably, carving out meaning from the smallest acts and thoughts, you can do the same as you concentrate on calming an arrhythmia or reducing the pain of angina. Directing your focus to your heart allows you to listen to it and pay attention to its needs, which you can supply.

How to Start a Stress Management Program

The hospital-based stress management programs like those of Drs. Ornish and Kabat-Zinn *require* group participation in these mind-body techniques, and comparisons between individuals who do and don't practice daily are startling—these techniques have as profound an effect on the recuperation process as diet and exercise. It has been found that the benefits of meditation, visualization, breathing, yoga, and tai chi are particularly valuable after a traumatic cardiac event to reduce the depression and anxiety that often follow a heart attack or bypass surgery.

If you have back or neck problems, check with your physician before doing any yoga or tai chi postures that might strain them. If you feel any discomfort while you are practicing either yoga or tai chi, or if you are short of breath, stop at once. Sit down and put your head between your knees, breathing calmly until your heart rate returns to normal. Start up your practice again only after resting for half an hour.

Yoga and tai chi are often taught at Ys and health clubs, and as college extension courses. You can ask at your local health food store or holistic health care center about classes, and also check your Yellow Pages under "Yoga," "Tai Chi Chuan," or "Martial Arts." There are also many corporations that now offer classes in both these disciplines and other stress management techniques as lunchtime options.

There are several good beginners' videotapes that can be useful, and books can serve as guides to the sequence of postures.

You'll need a quiet, open, well-ventilated space for your practice. If you're doing yoga, you'll need a mat with which to cushion the floor and a light blanket to cover yourself for the final ten minutes of the session. Work in loose, comfortable clothes. You may either go barefoot or wear sneakers or rope-soled slippers (available in Chinese markets) for tai chi.

Yoga

The practice of yoga (which means "yoke" or "union" in Sanskrit) dates back to the third century B.C., according to most sources. This meditative system of postures (called *asanas*) was developed in India as a means of unifying mind and body, using mental power to generate internal and external healing. These postures stretch, condition, and improve circulation to every part of you, and the breathing used in conjunction with them promotes relaxation and energy flow.

The stillness that you will start to feel at the end of one posture or a group of postures is a clue that you have tapped in to a new awareness of your own potential. If you can stay calm and alert through the petty annoyances and big problems of life, you have a new tool for alleviating stress and improving your heart health.

The yoga postures are held for different periods of time as you breathe into all parts of your body. Rather than thinking of holding on to anything, think instead of *releasing* into the posture. Although at first the poses may seem stiff and awkward, as you breathe into them, you will find that you can let go a little more, and then a little more.

As you become more skilled at assuming and moving through the postures, you will sense that your body is one whole, rather than an unrelated group of limbs and organs. You will unify all the structures of your body and be able to rally the strengths of healthy areas to compensate for the weaknesses you may have elsewhere.

Yoga benefits the heart and cardiovascular system because it stimulates a variety of tissues and glands that don't get massaged in conventional exercise or daily living. As you move and breathe more fully into a posture, you will trigger the secretion of hormones and neurotransmitters that will benefit both mind and body. The practice of yoga keeps the *prana,* or body's energy, in balance, which in turn keeps the entire cycle of mind and body in balance.

Yoga uses diaphragmatic breathing—that is, when you inhale, the stomach expands; when you exhale, the stomach contracts. This is the type of breathing used in most aerobic training and is really just an amplification of the natural breathing you do every day.

Yoga also employs several different types of directed breath work, and a particularly good one to promote relaxation is *alternate nostril breathing.* Place the thumb of your right hand on your right nostril and inhale, then exhale through your left. Then close off your left nostril with your fourth and fifth fingers and lift your thumb; inhale and exhale on the right side. This technique is not only centering, it also actively integrates right- and left-brain function, leaving you alert and calm.

To learn the basic postures, or *asanas,* it's best to join a yoga class taught by an experienced instructor. When you have a basic sequence that you can practice correctly in front of your teacher, you can work on your own without strain. There are many excellent audio- and videotapes on yoga that are readily available.

Tai Chi Chuan (Taijiquan)

This Chinese form of moving meditation offers not only a calm awareness of the spirit but the additional benefit of a flexible, strong body. The word *qi* (sometimes written *chi,* in Chinese transliteration, and *ki* in Japanese), means the same as *prana,* or "life force." The purpose of learning the grace-ful tai chi exercises or forms is to move the energy stored in the body to promote health and longevity. The movements of tai chi chuan, which means "grand ultimate fist," develop strength and flexibility as well as an ability to release and relax while moving. The ancillary breathing moves oxygen and energy throughout the body.

The type of breathing associated with Chinese medicine, known as *qi gong* (translated as "breath work"), has been used for centuries as a therapeutic technique. (See chapter 8 for a discussion of *qi gong* technique.)

Tai chi is based on the Taoist philosophy of nature that sees the universe as a balanced set of opposites. The *yin,* which stands for qualities of the earth, represents the yield-ing and responsive aspects of life; the *yang,* which stands for qualities of heaven, represents the strong and untiring as-pects. These two complementary forces are joined together and also contain within themselves the element of the other. We all have a little *yin* in our *yang;* we all have a little *yang* in our *yin.* They could not exist without each other.

The impact this concept has on healing is dramatic.

The combined opposites of yin and yang work in tai chi to teach you in a systematic way how to relax, how to focus and concentrate, and how to breathe so that your blood pressure and circulation are afforded the maximum benefits. As you move through the choreographed postures, or "forms," you are stimulating a variety of pressure points throughout your body (see chapter 8 for a discussion of acupoints and acupressure).

The internal massage offered by this type of practice is conceivably more valuable than the external exercise you get, although it is only by working internal and external together that you get the benefit of either one. As your mind becomes more flexible and yielding, accepting what you can and can't do physically, so your body becomes softer and more resilient.

The key to relaxation in tai chi is the idea of *sinking*. As you practice, you become magnetically bound to the floor. If you can master the feeling of letting go of your limbs, you can achieve a loose, relaxed body that is at the same time rooted and substantial.

There are documented cases of hypertensive individuals who, after two or three years of practice, no longer need medication to control their cholesterol or blood pressure. Very often arterial blockages in the legs that cause severe cramping (intermittent claudication) can be reduced or eliminated.

Because the tai chi forms are generally performed with bent legs, with the weight alternately shifting from one to the other, the practitioner develops a strong back and quadriceps, and blood flow to these areas increases. This often can take the burden off peripheral blood vessels in the lower legs that may have been constricted or narrowed.

The real bonus of tai chi for heart disease is the way in which both body and mind learn over time to let go and abandon stress. If medical science is correct in its relation of anger and tension to angina and heart attack, then this type of therapy removes the emotional triggers.

It's best to learn tai chi from a qualified instructor. Classes are widely available at Ys and health clubs around the country. Once you've learned a tai chi form, you can practice on your own without strain. There are also many excellent audio- and videotapes available.

Other Mind-Body Therapies

There are dozens of practitioners of mind-body therapies. The best-known and most widely practiced of these are the Alexander Technique and Feldenkrais Functional Integration and Awareness Through Movement. You will probably be able to find therapists who use these techniques through local holistic centers, YWCAs, or from notices on your health food store bulletin board.

Some of the other mind-body techniques may not be so easy to find, and yet the list keeps growing. You may wish to investigate Mari-EL Healing, One-Brain Therapy, Jin Shin Jyutsu, Rolfing, Polarity, Trager Psychophysical Integration, Hellerwork, Rubenfeld Synergy, Craniosacral Therapy, Transpersonal BodyMind therapy, and Reichian Breathwork, as well as various forms of massage.

Each of these therapies combines some type of exercise, manipulation, or laying on of hands with an exploration of inner tensions and blockages. The goal of all of them is to alleviate pain, improve general wellness, and provide stress relief. Some are aimed at healing specific areas of the mind and body and can be used to amplify the other complementary treatments you are receiving. Others may not be advisable for people with chronic heart conditions. You should check references carefully and talk to the clients of anyone who has "invented" his or her own therapeutic treatments.

Adding Another Link to the Chain of Holistic Care

The nature of complementary therapies is flexibility—one type of care amplifies another; one link in the chain supports all the others. As you are better able to handle stress in your life, your perspective and feelings will change. Your management of heart problems will become a part of management of your whole life.

The techniques outlined in this chapter require perseverance and dedication, yet they are deceptively simple in their healthful benefits. As you change your mind about your illness, you can make concrete differences in your body. One breath after another, one posture following the next, and slowly you will have a change of heart.

CHAPTER FIVE

What Supplementation Can Do for Heart Disease

If you are having an angina attack, or suddenly experience a bout of irregular heartbeats, taking a vitamin or mineral supplement will not offer immediate relief. Vitamins and minerals do have great preventive possibilities, however, and their benefit seems to increase the longer you take them. Even doctors and researchers who long scorned the idea of consuming vitamins for better health are now finding that appropriate supplementation can greatly augment the effects of medication for heart disease as well as other chronic conditions.

In addition to a daily multivitamin, those at risk for heart disease or who have already been diagnosed with the condition should consider a greater variety of vitamins, minerals, and the so-called quasi-vitamins and enzymes discussed in this chapter.

Consult your health care practitioner before taking any supplement, and be sure to discuss the ramifications of combining your medications with vitamins and minerals.

Getting Your Necessary Vitamins and Minerals

How can we get as many vitamins and minerals as we need in order to get well, stay well, and improve our cardiovascular system? Diet is the first and best source. You should be getting the majority of your nutrients from the meals you eat (see chapter 3) and only secondarily from the supplementation that supports a good diet.

However, it is exceptionally difficult to get all the vitamins and minerals you need to do the difficult job of healing tissue and boosting the immune system. For this reason, nutritionists and holistic practitioners generally advise some form of supplementation. The type and amount of supplement of course depend on your particular needs.

Vitamins

A vitamin is an organic substance that cannot be synthesized in the body. We take in vitamins from the food we eat, but some have to be ingested in precursor form and converted to the active substance by the body.

There are two types of vitamins: fat-soluble (A, D, E, and K) and water-soluble (all the Bs and C). The fat-soluble variety have to be carried on protein in the blood and are difficult to excrete. The water-soluble variety are more perishable and can be lost during storage and cooking. When they are ingested, they travel in the blood and lymph and are excreted in the urine. They can be stored only in limited amounts, unlike the fat-soluble ones, which are stored in the liver and fatty tissues of the body.

Minerals

Minerals are inorganic substances that remain after living plant or animal tissue is burned off. They work in conjunction with enzymes, hormones, and vitamins and help in nerve transmission, muscle contraction, cell permeability, tissue integrity and structure, protein metabolism, blood formation, energy production, and fluid regulation.

Minerals can work as partners, as a group endeavor, or they can be opponents in their work in the body; that is to say, some minerals enhance each other's absorption; some compete with each other for absorption.

Dosages and RDAs

How do we know which vitamins and minerals we need to improve a heart condition and which dosages to take? The RDAs (Required Daily Allowances) were originally set by the Food and Drug Administration as dosages below which the body would show a deficiency. The research on dosages for therapeutic benefit, however, is still in its infancy. Proponents of megadoses of vitamins are often thought of as charlatans, but no one yet knows how to get a healing effect from supplementation without experimenting at very high dosages.

Vitamin dosages are measured as either *mg* (milligrams), *mcg* (micrograms), or *IU* (international units). A milligram is a thousandth of a gram; a microgram is a thousandth of a milligram; an international unit is approximately 1.49 mg and is so designated because there has been an international agreement about the way to measure this particular substance. Note that the Recommended Daily Allowances from the U.S. Department of Agriculture are much lower than the recommended amounts for heart disease prevention.

Overdoses of vitamins are rare, but they do happen. Certain excessive amounts of fat-soluble vitamins (A and D) can be toxic; and megadoses of water-soluble Vitamin C can cause gastrointestinal upset. For this reason, stick to your personal daily recommended amounts of all supplements.

Which Supplements Should I Buy?

A health food store or mail-order catalog offers only "natural" varieties of supplements, which have no sugar, salt, preservatives, artificial colors, flavors, or sweeteners. They will also offer plant-based gelatin in their capsules, as opposed to the animal-based gelatins found in supermarket brands.

If you have already been diagnosed with heart disease, you should be very careful about everything you consume, which means you want to avoid additional salt in a daily vitamin supplement or a chemical binding agent that might conflict with a medication you are taking. So spending a little more for the natural brands is well worth it.

How to Start a Supplementation Program

Start by discussing your interest in supplementation with your primary-care physician. Many cardiologists and general-practice physicians are now interested in using vitamins and minerals as part of a complete cardiac care program.

If they are not expert in the field, however, they may refer you to a nutritionist who specializes in supplementation or to a hospital-based "heart-healthy" nutrition program. You can also consult the Resource Guide (chapter 11) for national organizations that can refer you to local practitioners.

The correct amounts for your condition must be set by your physician or health care practitioner, particularly if you are considering megadoses of any supplement.

Antioxidants Can Help Your Heart

Antioxidant protection has been proven effective against heart disease. Antioxidants are helpful substances—enzymes, vitamins, minerals, amino acids, and other compounds—that help to destroy "free radicals" in the body. Free radicals cause abnormal changes in cells that may lead to the development of heart disease and certain cancers. One of the ways in which free radicals do their harmful work is by using oxygen to alter LDL cholesterol. What occurs in the body is similar to the destructive process that turns fat rancid when left out in the open air.

Although our heart and bloodstream thrive on oxygen, it can also be a destructive gas. Oxidized cholesterol adheres to artery walls and hardens into atheromatous plaques, which makes it one of the chief culprits in heart disease.

But antioxidants, such as vitamins E, C, and beta-carotene, seem to be essential in maintaining healthy hearts because they deactivate free radicals and prevent them from destroying the molecular structure of our cells. They protect the delicate inner linings of blood vessels, which become increasingly susceptible to damage over the years. Antioxidants also help to strengthen cell walls so that free radicals can't invade.

A great deal of research on the value of antioxidants in the prevention and treatment of heart disease has been done over the past few years, and there are conflicting opinions. On the positive side we have much evidence that antioxidants are protective. One, an American study of nearly 12,000 individuals over ten years, showed that those taking the highest doses of vitamin C had a significant reduction in cardiac deaths (42 percent reduction for men; 25 percent for women). A vitamin E study done on twelve European groups showed that high blood levels of vitamin E correlated with low risk of heart attack deaths after accounting for other factors such as cholesterol and blood pressure levels. A study of 333 men with mild to moderate coronary artery disease who took beta-carotene for six years had half as many incidents of stroke, heart attack, sudden cardiac death, or the necessity for surgery as those taking a placebo.

On the negative side we have the recent study on Swedish smokers who took vitamins E, C, and beta-carotene and still ended up with lung cancer. Remember, however, that these individuals were exceptionally sick to begin with, and there has never been any claim that vitamin supplementation could reverse a chronic condition. It can, however, make a very big difference in helping to prevent heart disease.

Reducing Homocysteine Levels

Homocysteine (HCY) is a toxic amino acid, which we create by altering other amino acids that we make and ingest, such as those from pasteurized cow's milk and red meat. Homocysteine in turn helps to create arterial lesions.

A 1995 study came out with preliminary findings indicating that folic acid (available in dark leafy vegetables, whole grains, and kidney beans) significantly reduces homocysteine levels and may be able to reduce the risk of heart disease dramatically. It's been shown that supplements combining pyridoxine (vitamin B_6), choline, and folic acid can lower HCY by 32 percent in just three weeks. (Of course, cutting down on red meat and whole milk is also crucial!)

Which Vitamins Are Essential for Good Heart Health?

Multivitamins

Before you consider the larger amounts of individual nutrients mentioned below, you should protect yourself with a general, all-around multivitamin.

A very high-quality supplement would include a mix similar to the amounts listed below. These are between two and five times higher than the U.S. RDAs. If you are taking a multivitamin that has this elevated level of vitamin and mineral support, you will need to take much lower dosages of other supplements than the recommendations listed below:

Vitamin C	250 mg
Vitamin E	150 IU
Vitamin A	7,500 IU (one half from beta-carotene)
Iodine	150 mcg
Vitamin D	400 IU
Vitamins B_1, B_2, B_6, and niacin	75 mg each
Vitamin B_{12}	75 mcg
Calcium	50 mg
Potassium	10 mg
Iron	10 mg
Magnesium	7.2 mg
Manganese	6.1 mg
Zinc	15 mg
Selenium	10 mcg
Copper	0.5–1 mg
Chromium	25 mcg
Folic acid	400 mcg

Vitamin C (Ascorbic Acid)

Recommended protective amount: 1,000 mg daily.

Food sources: Broccoli, citrus fruits, tomatoes, and papaya. It is fairly easy to obtain all your vitamin C from food sources.

Risk of overdose: Large doses (over 3,000 mg) can cause nausea, diarrhea, and lower ability of white blood cells to fight foreign bacteria. If you have a history of forming oxalate kidney stones, overdosing on vitamin C could increase that tendency.

General information: Ascorbic acid is essential for cholesterol metabolism—it is responsible for the excretion of excess cholesterol from the body and is therefore a primary influence on the balance of good and bad lipids—one of the big factors in heart disease.

A report in the *American Journal of Clinical Nutrition* reported that the incidence of cardiovascular disease and cancer was lower in populations that consumed a diet high in vitamin C, with plenty of green leafy vegetables and fruit.

Vitamin E (Alpha, Beta, and Gamma Tocopherol)

Recommended protective amount: 400 to 800 IU daily.

Food sources: Olive oil, wheat germ, organ meats, and eggs. You will need supplementation since it would be fairly difficult to get your daily amount from food sources without eating a great deal of fat.

Risk of overdose: None documented in humans; however, large doses have been shown to cause growth retardation in animals.

General information: The tocopherol family protects fats from oxidizing in the body. It stabilizes membranes and keeps them from free-radical damage, helps maintain the structural integrity of skeletal, cardiac, and smooth muscle, and works with other antioxidants such as C and selenium to eradicate free radicals. It is also essential for the synthesis and maintenance of red blood cells.

The reason that vitamin E is so effective against cardiac problems is that it keeps one particular form of LDL cholesterol from oxidizing. It's the combination of this fat with oxygen that starts the chain of events leading to plaque deposits on the arteries.

Pigs on a diet high in vitamin E were found to have fewer

heart attacks. They were also able to recover from them more quickly than those who hadn't been given vitamins.

A 1994 study of American nurses, published in the *New England Journal of Medicine,* indicated that regular consumption of vitamin E lowered the risk of heart disease by 34 percent.

Vitamin E has also been used prior to bypass surgery to suppress the free radicals in the body during this traumatic procedure. Several patients, given 2,000 IU of vitamin E twelve hours before surgery, had no increase in free radicals, while the untreated patients had increasingly rising levels during and after their procedures.

Vitamin A (Retinol) and Its Precursor, Beta-carotene

Recommended protective amount of beta-carotene: 6.6 mg daily, or two carrots or one cantaloupe or two servings of squash.

Food sources: Carrots, squash, cantaloupe, tomatoes, dried fruits, fresh strawberries, broccoli, and brussels sprouts.

Risk of overdose: Over 50,000 IU of vitamin A daily can cause vomiting, weight loss, joint pain, itching, and cracked and bleeding lips. Excess beta-carotene may cause yellowish discoloration of the skin.

General information: Vitamin A and beta-carotene are essential for the maintenance of the epithelial tissue (all the mucous membranes in the body), and help to maintain elasticity in the tissues. Like vitamin E, beta-carotene also protects against the oxidizing of LDL cholesterol in the blood.

In a study of 1,300 subjects done at the Harvard Medical School, it was found that those who ate large amounts of beta-carotene had a significantly decreased mortality rate from cardiovascular disease when compared with a population who didn't eat much beta-carotene, after controlling all available cardiac risk factors. In another study of 333 men who had heart disease, those taking beta-carotene for six years had half as many heart attacks, strokes, incidence of sudden cardiac death, or bypass surgery as those on a placebo. A 1994 nurses' study showed that regular consumption of beta-carotene lowered the risk of heart disease by 22 percent.

Though recent reports downgrade the effectiveness of beta-carotene in preventing lung cancer in chronic smokers, other studies underline its effectiveness. In a six-year study on 22,000 physicians, researched at Brigham and Women's Hospital in Boston, those who were given beta-carotene supplements as opposed to a placebo had fewer heart attacks, strokes, and other cardiac events. The Physicians' Health Study showed that eating foods that contain beta-carotene can reduce the risk of stroke, heart attack, and death from cardiovascular disease by one half. In this study it was shown that beta-carotene prevented the oxidation of cholesterol—it is not able to stick to artery walls when it's not oxidized.

Niacin (Vitamin B₃, or Nicotinic Acid)

Recommended protective amount: 40 mg three times daily.

Food sources: Meat, fish, poultry, milk products, peanuts, and brewer's yeast—you can probably get your daily required amount from food without supplementation.

Risk of overdose: A niacin flush, where the skin becomes red and itchy, may occur, even at regular dosages. Prolonged use of more than 500 mg three times daily may cause high uric acid levels, elevated liver enzymes, and gastrointestinal problems. Do not take niacin if you have rheumatic heart disease or valve problems.

General information: Niacin takes part in over fifteen metabolic reactions, most of which are important in the release of energy from carbohydrates. It is also essential for fatty acid synthesis and oxidation of fatty acids. Niacin lowers the bad cholesterol, particularly the VLDLs (very-low-density lipoproteins) and triglycerides, while it raises good cholesterol (HDLs). It also balances blood sugar and dilates blood vessels, thereby improving circulation.

This vitamin has been shown to have enormous success in treatment of heart disease. Some physicians prescribe it in combination with a cholesterol-lowering drug such as lovastatin. However, since lovastatin reduces the body's ability to produce a heart-helper enzyme called CoQ10 (see page 107), you may want to ask your physician if you can take your niacin without any drugs. To avoid the typical "flush" that occurs when niacin is taken in doses over 75 mg over a long period of time, an aspirin a day is also recommended, or take niacin as inositol hexaniacinate.

It's important to be monitored carefully if you're taking a lot of niacin. Your doctor should check you periodically for high uric acid levels and elevated liver enzymes.

Pyridoxine (Vitamin B_6)

Recommended dosage for heart problems: 200 mg.

Food sources: Protein foods, such as meats and organ meats, poultry, fish, egg yolk, soybeans and dried beans, peanuts, and walnuts. You can also get it in bananas, avocados, cabbage, cauliflower, potatoes, whole grains, and prunes.

Risk of overdose: Some patients who are very sensitive may experience tingling and numbness in fingers at doses higher than 250 mg daily over time.

General information: This vitamin, important in protein breakdown and amino acid regulation, blocks the production of adenosine diphosphate (ADP), a by-product of the blood-clotting process. Vitamin B_6 acts as a cleanser and washes away the ADP, allowing freer blood circulation. Lipid, cholesterol, and carbohydrate metabolism are all dependent on having enough B_6.

Minerals That Protect Your Heart

Calcium

Recommended protective amount: 1,500 mg daily for women past menopause; 1,000 if they are taking replacement estrogen; 1,000 for men.

Food sources: Dairy products, green leafy vegetables, sea vegetables, and fish with bones. You may need supplementation unless you are willing to consume a great many green vegetables and fish with bones as well as low-fat or nonfat dairy products.

Risk of overdose: None. However, you should avoid dolomite and bone meal, which have been found to contain lead.

General information: Calcium is an important contributor to blood clotting and is used in the conversion of fibrinogen to fibrin. This mineral is also part of the makeup of blood platelets and plays a role in maintaining blood pressure. Because of its main function—preventing bone loss and keeping bone density high—it also helps an individual maintain an exercise program, which is part of the complete program of preventive heart care.

Magnesium

Recommended protective amount: 300 to 500 mg daily; the ratio should be half your calcium allowance.

Food sources: Green leafy vegetables, dry beans and peas, soybeans, nuts, whole grains.

Risk of overdose: Rare, except in individuals with kidney problems and those who abuse magnesium-based laxatives. They may experience drowsiness and weakness.

General information: Magnesium is necessary to activate an enzyme that helps transport potassium to the cells. If the body lacks sufficient magnesium, and the potassium balance is disturbed, arrhythmias may result. It's been found that there are fewer heart attacks in areas where magnesium levels in the drinking water are high.

Magnesium deficiencies appear to be significant in heart disease, heart attack, angina, stroke, arrhythmias, and hypertension. Magnesium, an electrolyte, keeps the balance of calcium and sodium low in the cells, particularly in the heart and blood vessels. Adequate magnesium ensures that the heart beats regularly, with the least stress possible. It helps to keep blood vessels expanded and relaxed, which lowers blood pressure.

Potassium

Recommended protective amount: 5 to 7 g daily.

Food sources: Bananas, potatoes, tomatoes, orange juice, apricots, lean meats, milk. Eating foods with a high-potassium–low-sodium ratio lowers the risk of heart attack and stroke. Bananas happen to have a 400:1 ratio; potatoes have a 200:1 ratio of these minerals.

Risk of overdose: Doses over 18 g may be toxic, resulting in cardiac dysfunction and kidney damage.

General information: Potassium, which is found primarily in the intracellular fluids of the body, helps maintain cell integrity and water balance. It is also essential for muscle contraction, glycogen formation, and carbohydrate metabolism. Potassium is also an electrolyte and helps to maintain the heart's electrical impulses and adequate heart rate.

Chromium Picolinate

Recommended protective amount: Up to 200 mcg daily.

Food sources: Brewer's yeast, meat, cheese, cereals, whole grains, but only if unprocessed. Eating a lot of sugar will deplete your chromium supplies.

Risk of overdose: Long-term doses over 500 mcg daily may inhibit insulin activity.

General information: Chromium picolinate reduces LDLs

and total cholesterol and keeps blood sugar in balance. This mineral works with insulin in the body to regulate carbohydrate and lipid metabolism. It allows the body to increase HDLs, which act as scavengers in the blood, searching out LDL cholesterol and returning it to the liver for processing. It can also strip bad cholesterol deposits from the arteries, which in turn would reduce the incidence of plaque. It also increases the utilization and effectiveness of niacin. When chromium is combined with picolinic acid, a natural metal chelator (see chapter 9 for an explanation of chelation), it makes chromium more available for absorption. Adding chromium to the diet helps the insulin to get cholesterol out of the bloodstream more quickly, before it can oxidize and damage blood vessel walls.

Selenium

Recommended protective amount: 200 to 400 mcg. This trace mineral generally comes packaged with vitamin E.

Food sources: Meats, fish, cabbage, mushrooms, onions, whole grains. It is found in the soil in almost all areas.

Risk of overdose: Amounts over 400 mcg may be toxic and can cause liver disease and heart abnormalities.

General information: Selenium appears to boost the potential of vitamin E as an antioxidant to keep cell integrity. It protects cell membranes from oxidation damage and fibrosis.

Quasi-Vitamins and Enzymes—New Hope for Better Hearts

Coenzyme Q-10 (CoQ10)

Recommended protective amount for heart patients: 120 to 360 mg daily; recommended protective dosage for healthy individuals, 10 to 30 mg daily.

Food sources: Beef, sardines, spinach, and peanuts, as well as organ meats such as heart, kidney, and liver.

Risk of overdose: None documented.

This coenzyme, also known as ubiquinone, is actually a vitamin that appears to regulate the flow of oxygen in the cells and helps in the body's production of adenosine triphosphate (ATP), which supplies a biochemical "spark" that creates cellular energy in the body. CoQ10 also has antioxidant properties, so it protects cells from free-radical damage. When we take in CoQ10, it immediately concentrates in the heart muscle.

The body produces its own supply of this "vitamin" if it has sufficient amounts of vitamins B_2, B_3, B_6, folic acid, pantothenic acid, and vitamin C. But most Americans don't eat a sufficiently well-balanced diet to get all these essential nutrients, which means they aren't producing enough CoQ10 to help their hearts.

Nearly all forms and symptoms of heart disease—heart failure, mitral valve prolapse, hypertension, enlarged heart, angina, ischemic heart disease (reduced blood flow)—seem to respond well to supplemental CoQ10.

More and more frequently CoQ10 is being used sucessfully as a treatment for angina. It improves heart function, even in cases of severe cardiac disease. In a six-year study at the University of Texas, 806 congestive-heart-failure patients took CoQ10, and 75 percent of them survived for three years, as compared with only 25 percent who survived with conventional therapy. When this coenzyme was given to people with hypertension, their blood pressures dropped significantly, even *without* using medication or diet.

There are many cases of individuals with heart failure who have done poorly on medication who appear to thrive on CoQ10. Their enlarged hearts reduce in size and begin pumping normally. They are able to go from lives as sedentary invalids to thriving, active people.

In therapy it is typically used for six to twelve months, at which point many heart patients find their condition is so improved, their physicians reduce the dosages of their medications. A side issue to this is that lovastatin, a drug typically used to reduce cholesterol, inhibits the production of CoQ10, as do several of the beta-blockers used for hypertension. This is yet another reason to select a knowledgeable holistic doctor who can weigh the benefits of both and help you decide which is right for you.

Lysine

Recommended protective amount: 500 mg daily on an empty stomach.

Food sources: Milk.

Risk of overdose: None, but more effective if you do not eat seeds, nuts, peas, and chocolate.

General information: This amino acid is particularly beneficial for those with atherosclerosis because it makes a particular type of cholesterol known as Lp(a), or ''lipoprotein little a,'' less sticky. It also metabolizes into L-carnitine, which suppresses formation of lactic acid that some experts feel may be partly responsible for heart attacks.

L-carnitine

Recommended protective amount: 500 to 1,000 mg daily.

Food sources: Tempeh, tofu, beef, lamb, avocado.

Risk of overdose: Do not take over 1,600 mg daily over a period of a year without consulting a nutrition specialist.

General information: This amino acid transports fatty acids into the part of the cell necessary to burn fats for energy—the mitochondria—and is therefore responsible for keeping the heart and other muscles vital. It reduces triglyceride levels and raises HDLs. Because carnitine stimulates the breakdown of long-chain fatty acids, which are the preferred energy source in well-oxygenated heart tissue, supplementation is often beneficial, particularly if you have already been diagnosed with heart disease. Individuals who don't have good oxygen supply in their blood require more carnitine.

Because this vitaminlike compound is so effective against angina and atherosclerosis, it's been found that some patients on beta-blockers, calcium channel blockers, and nitrates need less medication after carnitine supplementation.

Lecithin

Recommended protective amount: 2 capsules or 1 tablespoon with meals, taken with vitamin E, which speeds its assimilation into the body.

Food sources: Used as an emulsifying agent in many foods (see labels).

Risk of overdose: None.

General information: Lecithin, which is mostly composed of the vitamin choline, contains linoleic acid and inositol. It is a fatty substance (although it acts as a fat emulsifier in the blood) that is a part of all cell membranes. Because it helps to keep the membranes elastic and flexible, it is useful in the treatment of atherosclerosis.

Plant Enzymes

Recommended protective amount: None set.

Food sources: Soy products (tempeh, tofu, miso).

Risk of overdose: None.

General information: These fungal enzymes are derived from *Aspergillus oryzae*. They appear to be easier for the body to assimilate than those derived from animal sources and have been used successfully to treat chronically obstructed arteries. *A. oryzae* seems to be much more effective than heparin, an anticoagulant, in improving blood flow through stiff arterial segments.

In a 1978 study eighteen patients with intermittent claudication (a painful condition resulting from insufficient blood supply to the legs) were given either *A. oryzae* or an anticoagulant and placebo for three months. The anticoagulant produced no changes; however, the enzyme significantly improved circulation in over half the obstructed arterial segments in the patients.

Pycnogenol

Recommended protective amount: 30 mg daily.

Food sources: Fruits, vegetables, and other plants such as grapes, cranberries, beans, and cola nuts. As a supplement, it is made from the bark of a European coastal pine tree or from grape seed.

Risk of overdose: None.

General information: Pycnogenol is a powerful antioxidant that protects the good qualities of vitamin C and makes sure that the vitamin isn't oxidized as it is absorbed.

Pycnogenol is a bioflavonoid, or botanical element that has estrogenic qualities, and strengthens the circulatory system.

This bioflavonoid helps to reduce blood vessel damage and inflammation, as well as other free-radical damage. It protects the blood platelets and doesn't allow them to clump together and form clots that might result in blockages. It also keeps the platelets from adhering to arterial walls. Pycnogenol doesn't just protect, it actually improves the condition of arteries and capillaries by stabilizing the collagen (protein) involved in repair and regrowth of tissues.

Essential Fatty Acids (EFAs)

LINOLEIC ACID

Recommended protective amount: None set.

Food sources: Safflower, corn, and sunflower oils. Unfortunately processing converts much of the fatty acids in these oils to unusable forms.

Risk of overdose: None.

General information: Linoleic acid is valuable to the body after it is converted to GLA (gamma-linoleic acid), which converts again during an enzyme process before forming prostaglandins.

Prostaglandins are hormonelike substances that are influential in many different biological activities, including the functioning of the heart and cardiovascular system. The twenty or so prostaglandins that have been identified so far cannot be stored, but are made as needed by the cells—one is a powerful anticlotting agent. By keeping platelets from clumping together, prostaglandins help to retard plaque buildup on artery walls.

EFAMOL (also known as EVENING PRIMROSE OIL)

Recommended protective amount: 500 mg twice daily.

Food sources: None.

Risk of overdose: None.

General information: The evening primrose plant contains gamma-linoleic acid, so when you consume the oil, your body gets GLA directly. Efamol has proved effective in lowering blood pressure in hypertensive patients, in lowering serum cholesterol, and in reducing the risk of thrombosis. Women at risk for estrogen-dependent cancers may wish to substitute borage oil or black currant oil to get GLA directly.

EPA (EICOSAPENTAENOIC ACID)

Recommended protective amount: 1,000 to 2,000 mg daily of a marine-lipid concentrate such as Max EPA (daily supplements of 5–10 g) or SuperEPA.

Food sources: Cold saltwater fatty fishes, such as cod, mackerel, and herring.

Risk of overdose: EPA should be avoided completely by individuals on anticoagulant medications.

General information: This omega-3 fatty acid has been shown to lower serum cholesterol levels, decrease triglycerides, control arterial spasms, and prevent the production of blood clots.

Fish oils, like linoleic acid, are also precursors to prostaglandins. The more EPA in the diet, therefore, the greater the ability on the part of the cells to produce these beneficial clot-busting substances.

These good omega-3 fats are predominant in the diet of Eskimos and Japanese. Although a recent study on doctors who consumed fish once a week attempted to disprove the theory that eating fish is good for your heart, the problem may lie in the amount of fish oils taken in. A higher dosage than what eating salmon once a week can provide is probably needed for cardiovascular health.

So when your mother made you take your cod liver oil every morning, she was actually helping to prevent heart disease in your adult life! In one study, volunteers took 50 grams of cod liver oil daily for twenty-three days. Serum cholesterol declined in most subjects by 27 percent, and rose rapidly when the cod liver oil treatment was discontinued.

Supplementation as a Way of Life

Although heart disease is the biggest killer in our country, the numbers of heart attacks and strokes have actually declined since 1965—just about the time that the American public came to a new awareness of how an excellent diet can supply vitamins and minerals that will truly protect the heart. Supplementation came out of the closet at about this time as well and was no longer the fad of a few "health nuts." Ongoing research about the potential of vitamins and quasi-vitamins, minerals, and enzymes will undoubtedly influence our heart health greatly in the decades to come.

Unlike medication, vitamins and minerals take a long time to make changes in the body. This means that if you are at risk for heart disease or have already been diagnosed with the condition, and wish to protect yourself with supplementation, you must commit to a long-term program supervised by your holistic practitioner or a licensed nutritionist.

CHAPTER SIX

What Herbs Can Do for Your Heart

Herbal medicine is probably the oldest form of healing on earth. In this chapter we will explore the uses of botanical medicine for heart disease as well as for protecting and supporting a healthy cardiovascular system.

Herbal therapy is incredibly versatile—you can use the flowers, leaves, roots, rhizomes, bark, and seeds of plants to heal in a multitude of different ways. You can make a tea, decoction, or infusion of the plant and drink it, distill it in alcohol for a tincture or extract, turn it into a salve or cream for a topical application, soak in an herbal preparation in a bath, or you can capture its essence by inhaling it (aromatherapy) in order to get its medicinal effects.

Although there are wonderful advantages to botanical medicine for heart disease, these natural compounds are potent substances and should be used with caution. Herbs can be harmful—even lethal—if used improperly, and they therefore must be carefully prescribed and dosed. **Always consult your health care practitioner before using any herbal preparation.**

Plants that are medicinally useful contain active compounds that either promote certain reactions or inhibit certain processes in our cells. But rather than attempt to heal the body by concentrating on only one chemical element—as a drug does—plants heal by using many compounds in combination to affect every system of the body.

Our ancestors, using family and tribal traditions as well as experimentation, gathered and prepared herbs in different ways to treat different conditions. They learned at what times of year a certain plant had the most benefit—when it was flowering, for example, or when its poisonous berries had dropped off. They discovered the best ways to get many uses from one plant—eating the plant, rubbing the leaves on a wound, boiling the bark or cut-up roots. They found some plants to be calming, while others stimulated; some were antiseptic, anti-inflammatory, analgesic, sedative, styptic, antibiotic, hallucinogenic, tonic, or cleansing.

The debate still rages as to whether to use the whole plant or one active ingredient of the plant when treating a condition. The traditional school says that it is important to include everything when considering an herb for medicinal use—that various elements offset others that might be dangerous and that the combination works on the total body rather than just the affected organ or tissue. The more scientific approach states that it's safer to remove the toxic elements and use only those parts that are appropriate for healing. The "whole plant" theory, of course, is more in line with the thinking of holistic medicine—you must consider a balance of elements in order to reap the true benefits of the remedies.

Unless you are very knowledgeable about picking, preparing, and using herbs, it's best to rely on the herbal companies mentioned in the Resource Guide (see chapter 11) to sell you ready-to-use preparations of healing herbs. The plant extracts you'll buy are standardized with reliable dosage delivery of active ingredients.

Why Plants Heal

A plant is composed of multiple components, such as proteins, enzymes, sugars, fats, hormonal precursors, vitamins, and minerals, that protect and nourish the plant and may also affect the humans or animals who use it. Certain properties of a plant can keep it safe from bacteria and fungi that might threaten to kill it; those same properties, when ingested as a tea, can ward off bacteria that might prove harmful to the human body.

The various active elements in herbs

- are cardiotonic; that is, they make the heart pump more efficiently by binding to heart muscle and increasing each contraction without increasing the heart's need for oxygen.
- are diuretic; that is, they allow the kidneys to excrete salt and water. Normally urine output is two thirds to three quarters of your daily fluid intake. However, with botanical diuretic therapy, the body will excrete as much liquid as it takes in, while retaining vital nutrients, vitamins, and minerals.
- are hypotensive; that is, they relax the blood vessels, moderating the force of blood pumped against the arterial walls during each contraction.
- are tonic; that is, they nourish and support the body as a whole, as opposed to just one organ or system.

What Is a Tonic?

In centuries past, mothers used to offer various "tonics" to their children as "something that's good for what ails you." The concept of a tonic goes back to herbal therapy, however.

Any mixture of herbs gives you a combination of different

components, such as vitamins, minerals, hormonal precursors, and enzymes. This means that in addition to the main action you receive from the herb, you get many other supportive factors that are good for your system (as opposed to a drug such as an antibiotic, which often cures the immediate problem but depletes the system).

Tonics, then, will treat an acute problem and a chronic one simultaneously. They work directly on the target organ and also improve the overall functioning of the whole body slowly over a period of months.

For example, a person with high blood pressure needs an herb that is hypotensive and will lower pressure. But since the high blood pressure may be caused by excess fluid (kidney imbalance), liver congestion, poor heart function, and poor peripheral circulation, you need herbs to correct these problems and also nourish and restore sound organ function to the system that may be the underlying cause of the condition. Tonics also act preventively, keeping systems strong so that they don't break down.

Certain herbs serve a variety of functions: Broom is used to *raise* blood pressure in cases of heart failure, whereas motherwort will *lower* blood pressure and reduce the pain of angina.

When beginning herbal therapy, it's best to start slowly, with a heart tonic—garlic would help the heart and all other systems simultaneously. Then, depending on your symptoms, you might add the classic heart tonic hawthorn; a stimulant such as cayenne; a nervine such as valerian; or a diuretic like dandelion leaf once in a while, taking small amounts one at a time.

Reaping the Benefits of Herbs in Conventional Medicine

Many of the medicines we get in the drugstore today are refined or synthetic versions of plant substances. Modern pharmacology subtracts the harmful elements from plants and purifies the results down to one specific constituent. (One advantage of the single compound is that all possible toxins are removed from the original mix.)

Digoxin, the medication derived from digitalis, is a refined and synthesized form of the foxglove plant. In 1766, an English physician named William Withering came upon a "wisewoman" who had been dosing clients with potent herbal concoctions that made them feel better. He paid her handsomely for packets of these mysterious herbs, only one of which proved to have healing powers: This was foxglove, a heart stimulant.

Withering performed numerous scientific tests on the powder he made from this herb, which he called digitalis. He found that the medicine caused heart muscles to contract strongly and briskly, staving off cardiac insufficiency. The improved timing of contractions gave the heart more opportunity to rest between beats and enabled it to deliver blood to the rest of the circulatory system at a lower pressure.

Foxglove should never be used in herbal therapy; the active ingredients—steroidal substances known as cardiotonic glycosides—can be lethal. However, the plant is useful in conventional medicine because of the drug produced from it. By working intracellularly on potassium and sodium levels, these particular glycosides increase the action of calcium on muscles—which causes all the muscles in the body, including the heart, to contract more powerfully. These compounds can be extracted and processed as the medication digoxin in order to regulate heart rate.

But when you use a plant to heal the body, you are employing an arsenal of biologically active compounds, which work together to effect change. Because herbs offer many different properties from one source, you are more likely to derive some good (without so many side effects) from botanical medicine than from a pharmaceutical product. Even if you are only taking an herb to help one symptom, you are at the same time getting extra benefits: possibly a tonic, or a diuretic, or a sweat-inducing effect as well. The difference between herbal healing and medication has been compared to the difference between buckshot, which sprays out a volley against the enemy, and a single "magic bullet" that has a very specific direction.

It's interesting to compare the effects of the drug digitalis, which is refined from a plant, with the unadulterated herb hawthorn berry.

The most "classic" heart herb is hawthorn. A small study conducted in 1984 showed that hawthorn tablets reduced angina by 84 percent as compared with only a 37 percent reduction with a placebo. Of the twenty-nine patients taking hawthorn, thirteen of them were able to stop taking their nitroglycerine tablets, and another ten reduced their dosage and frequency of the medication. Hawthorn improves heart circulation by dilating the blood vessels and increasing oxygenation. It also normalizes and nourishes the total circulatory function.

Both hawthorn and digitalis dilate the coronary arteries and peripheral blood vessels; they both lower blood pressure and reduce the burden placed on the heart; they both maximize oxygen uptake by the heart during exercise; and they both increase enzyme metabolism in the heart muscle, which makes for a stronger cardiovascular system.

However, hawthorn contains no cardiotonic glycosides, as digitalis does, and therefore does not have any of the adverse toxic effects of digitalis, which include nausea, blurred vision, headache, drowsiness, arrhythmias, and sometimes death. The herb acts directly on the heart and also on other organs that affect circulation, such as the kidneys, liver, and peripheral vessels, so it lowers blood pressure in a more indirect and therefore safer manner than digitalis does. It also works to support the healthy heart; it doesn't just work on muscle fiber in the heart, as digitalis does. Hawthorn berry also performs as a tonic, enhancing cardiac output.

If you're currently taking medication, you may wish to complement and enhance the effect of drugs with herbal therapy but you *must* do so under careful medical supervision. If you are not taking drugs, herbs can provide a suitable nourishing tonic to help keep your heart in the best shape possible.

How to Buy and Prepare Herbs

If you have a garden, you can always be sure of fresh herbs. You should have an excellent knowledge of horticulture before you attempt to use fresh herbs for medicinal purposes, however. The most common use of herbs is one in which the dried roots, bark, leaves, flowers, or berries are steeped in water and the resulting liquid is consumed.

But for those who haven't got time for this, the easiest way to take herbs is in a ready-to-use form. There are also freeze-dried varieties, usually packed in capsules, which will stay potent much longer than the dried version. You can also take your herbs as an extract (the essential oil that has been extracted from the plant), or as a tincture (a plant extract dissolved in alcohol). And there are gels and creams, for topical use.

It's best to buy dried herbs in the amount you need so that your herbs stay fresh. Once dried and exposed to light, herbs lose their potency. After six months, loose herbs are virtually worthless, so it's better to buy in small quantities.

Be sure you are buying from a reputable source, such as

the mail-order companies listed in the Resource Guide (chapter 11). You want to be sure that you are getting the pure herb that has been harvested at the right time and processed correctly. Your best bet is to buy organic domestic herbs that have not been sprayed with chemicals. Avoid imported varieties that haven't been tested in this country.

You can use herbs in a variety of forms (it is not essential to take them with food unless that is specified on the label of the herb you purchase):

- AS A TEA: Put 1 heaping teaspoon of dried herb in a tea ball, immersed in 1 cup of hot water. Teas made in this way are usually too weak to give medicinal benefits; however, they are very helpful as a daily tonic.

  For stronger medicinal effect, you should consider the infusions, decoctions, capsules, and tinctures.

- AS AN INFUSION: Place 1 ounce of flowers and leaves in a pint jar, cover with boiling water, and allow to steep. Steep leaves for 4 hours, flowers for 2, and seeds for ½ hour. Drink two cups (16 ounces) of infusion per day if you weigh from 125 to 150 pounds; three cups daily if you weigh from 150 to 200 pounds; four cups if over 200 pounds. If the taste is too bitter, you may sweeten with a little juice.

- AS A DECOCTION: This is an infusion made from hard roots, bark, or seeds. Use the same proportions as the infusion, bring to a boil, and simmer for ten to 15 minutes. You can boil them longer to reduce the amount of liquid, but you will lose lots of essential vitamins and minerals that way.

- AS A CAPSULE: Depending on the herb and the size of the capsule, take two to three capsules, twice or three times daily. You should purchase freeze-dried extracts of plants packed into gelatin capsules.

- AS A TINCTURE: Depending on the particular herb and the concentration of the tincture, take ½ to 1 teaspoon, twice or three times daily in ¼ cup of water. (If you put them in boiled water, this decreases the alcohol content.) Shake the bottle well before filling the dropper. (An extract or tincture is prepared by soaking fresh or dried herbs in an alcohol solution. There are alcohol-free, glycerin-based extracts available as well.)
- IN AROMATHERAPY: Place 2 drops of specified essential oil in a vaporizer or bath; or mix with 1 teaspoon carrier oil (sweet almond, wheat germ, or grape seed oil) topically for massage.

Dosages

Herbs are synergistic; that is, all the properties of one particular herb enhance each separate property. If you take several herbs in combination, the effects of some of these herbs will be enhanced. Certain herbs are contraindicated during pregnancy and others if you have chronic hypertension. (All cautions for the herbs discussed in this chapter are mentioned within their listing.) Remember that a small dose of a certain herb may do nothing to affect your condition, but a large dose of the same herb could aggravate it or even worsen it.

The dosage varies with the particular herb, but most experts counsel you to take 5 to 30 drops (½ to 1 teaspoon) of tincture or 2–4 cups of infusion or two capsules three times daily.

How to Start an Herbal Treatment Program

As preventive medicine, herbal therapy will strengthen and support your cardiovascular system as well as all the other systems in your body. If you have already been diagnosed with heart disease or any other specific medical condition, you will need to discuss with your health care provider whether long-term herbal therapy is advisable for your particular condition, and whether you can mix herbs with your allopathic medicines.

You should begin, under a naturopathic physician's or an herbalist's supervision, with low dosages of single herbs (see Resource Guide, chapter 11, for a referral). You should also find a good health food store with a knowledgeable owner who can direct you to the herbs you need.

What follows is a listing of the herbs you might use to treat the various problems of heart disease.

Herbs Frequently Used for Heart Disease

Tonics

HAWTHORN *(Crategus oxyacantha)*, also called Mayblossom, Whitethorn

Hawthorn is the quintessential "heart herb." Because it enhances cardiac output, it acts directly on the heart, but also on other organs that affect circulation, such as the kidneys, liver, and peripheral vessels.

Parts used: Flowers, leaves, berries.

Properties: Vasodilator; ability to regulate blood pressure and heart irregularities; lowers blood serum cholesterol levels.

Indications: High or low blood pressure; heart and circulatory problems. It will take about three months of daily herb therapy to see results.

GARLIC *(Allium sativum)*

Garlic contains several active sulfur compounds, one of which is *allicin.* This compound blocks the biosynthesis of cholesterol. Dietary garlic also helps to expand blood vessel walls, allowing for enhanced blood flow. This lowers blood pressure. Another chemical in garlic, *ajoene,* keeps blood vessels from sticking together and may help to prevent clots.

Garlic is most potent when eaten raw; you can chop it and sprinkle it on your food, using one or two cloves daily. You can also take odorless garlic pills (Kyolic).

Parts used: Bulb, cloves.

Properties: Antibacterial, hypotensive.

Indications: High blood pressure; high blood serum cholesterol levels.

Diuretics

YARROW *(Achillea millefolium)*, **also called Milfoil, Woundwort, Carpenter's Weed**

Yarrow is an effective diuretic in that it gets the body to sweat and rids it of toxins. By dilating peripheral blood vessels, yarrow also helps to lower blood pressure and at the same time tones the blood vessels.

Parts used: Whole plant in flower.

Properties: Diuretic, diaphoretic (sweat-inducing), hypotensive.

Indications: Hypertension; coronary thrombosis.

CAUTION: Not for long-term use. Large doses may cause headaches and dizziness.

DANDELION *(Taraxacum officinale)*, also called Pee in the Bed, Lion's Teeth, Fairy Clock

Dandelion leaf is a diuretic and kidney tonic with supportive iron and magnesium. Dandelion root is a liver tonic. Both stimulate the release of digestive enzymes and filter toxins and wastes from the bloodstream, allowing the body to excrete them. Since a healthy liver and kidneys are prerequisites to eliminating toxins, it is interesting to note that dandelion also relieves chronic liver congestion and helps the kidney to get rid of excess fluid.

Parts used: Fresh or dried root, leaves, and flowers.

Properties: Bitter tonic, liver drainer, diuretic.

Indications: Fluid retention; the need to build up the body (dandelion has high potassium content).

PARSLEY *(Petroselinum crispum)*

Parsley is a wonderful diuretic, but at the same time it is high in vitamin C content, thereby restoring much-needed nutrients to the body.

Parts used: Taproot, leaves, seeds.

Properties: Diuretic, expectorant.

Indications: Fluid retention; general need to build up the body.

CAUTION: Do not use during pregnancy in medicinal doses.

YELLOW DOCK *(Rumex crispus)*, also called Curled Dock, Rumex

This herb is known for its high iron content, so it's used in the treatment of anemia. It also affects the liver and related organs so that they can better purify the blood.

Parts used: Rootstock, young leaves.

Properties: Liver and gallbladder tonic, laxative, iron supplement.

Indications: Anemia; the need for a general tonic for whole system.

BURDOCK ROOT *(Arctium lappa)*

Burdock is an overall blood cleanser, removing toxins from the body via the urine and sweat. It also enhances liver and bile functions.

Parts used: Fresh or dried roots, seeds (leaves are toxic).

Properties: Diuretic, diaphoretic, laxative, antimicrobial, bitter tonic, liver drainer (encourages secretion of bile).

Indications: Arthritis, liver congestion.

CAUTION: To be used only under supervision during pregnancy.

Hypotensives (Lower Blood Pressure)

LIME BLOSSOM *(Tilia cordata, Tiliaceae)*

Lime, also known as linden (American basswood), has been used for centuries in eastern European medicine to lower high blood pressure. The volatile oil of this plant contains glycosides and manganese salts in addition to other constituents.

Parts used: Bark, fresh leaves, flowers.

Properties: Hypotensive, antispasmodic.

Indications: Hypertension (used in combination with hawthorn).

CAUTION: Excessive use of this tea is contraindicated.

Peripheral Vasodilator (Dilates Blood Vessels)

GINGKO *(Gingko biloba),* also called Hill Apricot, Silver Fruit, Pak-Ko (Chinese)

This extremely safe herb dates back to the dinosaurs, and although it is typically thought of as a dilator of blood vessels in the brain, it is generally good for circulatory problems throughout the body. Like hawthorn, gingko is most effective when taken over several months.

Parts used: Leaves, fruits, nuts.

Properties: Vasodilator, antioxidant, improves circulation, reduces peripheral edema, improves blood vessel tone.

Indications: Stroke, nervous system disorders, peripheral circulatory problems.

Circulatory Stimulants

GINGER *(Zingiber officinale)*

Ginger, native to both India and China, has been used medicinally for thousands of years. It produces a feeling of warmth and alertness and appears to have antioxidant properties, since it retards fat spoilage in meat.

Parts used: Fresh or dried rhizome.

Properties: Stimulant, carminative (gas-producing).

Indications: Poor circulation; flatulence; spasms.

CAUTION: Excessive use may cause or exacerbate skin irritations.

GINSENG *(Eleutherococcus senticosus)*, also called Siberian Ginseng

Ginseng, or "manroot" in Chinese, refers to three different plants that often have the basic human shape. The Asian and American varieties both have many health-giving properties; however, Siberian ginseng is most appropriate for individuals with heart disease.

Parts used: Dried root.

Properties: Stimulant.

Indications: The need for revitalization, feelings of lethargy and fatigue; high or low blood pressure.

CAUTION: Large doses may have the same effect as too much caffeine and may cause nervousness and insomnia. Should not be combined with caffeinated beverages.

PRICKLY ASH BARK *(Zanthoxylum americanum)*, also called Toothache Tree

Prickly ash bark is a nervous system stimulant. It contains alkaloids, lignans, and other substances that may trigger glandular secretions.

Parts used: Dried stem and root bark.

Properties: Circulatory stimulant, diaphoretic, expectorant.

Indications: The need to revitalize the system—the herb gives a warm glow, a sense of nervous tingling, almost an "electric" feeling.

CAYENNE *(Capsicum frutescens)*, also called Tabasco, Pepper

Capsaicin, the active constituent of cayenne, prevents a rise in liver cholesterol levels and also reduces blood pressure. Because it is diaphoretic, it stimulates the body to get rid of toxins by sweating. As it promotes cardiovascular activity, it also lowers blood pressure.

Parts used: Dried ground fruit.

Properties: Stimulant, antiseptic.

Indications: Poor peripheral circulation; absorption of cholesterol; high blood pressure.

CAUTION: Large doses are extremely irritating to the gastrointestinal system.

Nervines (Antistress)

MOTHERWORT *(Leonurus cardiaca)* also called Heart Wort, Heart Gold, Heart Heal

Due to its high glycoside and alkaloid content, motherwort is an excellent heart tonic. It calms palpitations and normalizes heart function when taken in small doses.

Parts used: Fresh or dried flowering plant.

Properties: Sedative, cardiotonic, hypotensive.

Indications: Anxiety; tachycardia.

CAUTION: Potentially toxic in large doses. May cause dermatitis if rubbed on skin.

St. John's Wort *(Hypericum perforatum)*

St. John's wort is very useful for menopausal women who may also be suffering from anxiety, or from rheumatic or neuralgic pain. It is not recommended for serious clinical depression, however.

Parts used: Fresh or dried flowering plant tops, fresh flowers.

Properties: Antidepressant, anti-inflammatory, antiviral.

Indications: Depression, anxiety, poor blood circulation.

CAUTION: This herb has been shown to cause skin sensitivity to sunlight in animal studies.

Valerian *(Valeriana officinalis)*, also called Setwall

One of the most studied of all plants, valerian root and its constituents, the valepotriates, have sedative, hypotensive, and tranquilizing effects on higher brain centers. This herb has no side effects. You can use a dropperful or up to one teaspoonful in water at night if you have trouble sleeping; use half of that as a daytime calmant.

Parts used: Root.

Properties: Sedative, nervine.

Indications: Nervous tension, aggressive tendencies, insomnia, headaches, hypertension.

CAUTION: Some people experience a stimulating rather than a sedative effect from valerian.

Skullcap *(Scutellaria laterifolia)*, also called Helmet Flower, Mad-Dogweed, Virginian Scullcap

In addition to being a nerve tonic, skullcap improves circulation and strengthens the heart muscle.

Parts used: Aerial parts.

Properties: Tonic for nervous system, sedative.

Indications: Anxiety, depression, insomnia, nervous headaches, stress, hypertension.

Antispasmodics

CRAMPBARK *(Viburnum opulum)*, also called Guelder Rose, Highbush Cranberry Bark

Crampbark acts as a muscle relaxant, but is also good for any type of uterine or ovarian pain or bleeding.

Parts used: Dried stem bark.

Properties: Sedative, spasmolytic.

Indications: Muscle spasms; bleeding associated with menopause.

CAUTION: The fresh berries are poisonous.

Other Herbs That Might Be Used for Heart Disease

An herbalist may decide that your real problem is not the heart itself, but rather other systems that affect the heart. Therefore you might be prescribed bugleweed to regulate a thyroid problem or if you have diabetes; you might take black cohosh if you had any condition where you suffered cramps, such as arthritis or menopausal joint pains.

BUGLEWEED *(Lycopus virginicus)*, also called Virginia Bugleweed

Bugleweed acts specifically to regulate a hyperactive thyroid gland, particularly if there are palpitations, shaking, and difficulty breathing.

Parts used: Fresh or dried flowering plant.

Properties: Sedative.

Indications: High pulse rate in conditions involving overactive thyroid gland; diabetes.

BLACK COHOSH *(Cimicifuga racemosa),* also called Black Snakeroot, Bugbane

This herb is believed to contain several resins that inhibit the vasomotor centers in the central nervous system. This allows for better dilation of blood vessels and a lowering of pressure.

Parts used: Dried rootstock.

Properties: Hypotensive, vasodilator, sedative, antispasmodic, contains phytoestrogens (plant estrogens).

Indications: Cramping, high blood pressure, anxiety, high cholesterol.

CAUTION: Large doses irritate nerve centers; may cause uterine contractions—therefore, **in pregnancy this should be used only during the last four weeks, and only with a physician's approval.**

Treatment by Condition or Symptom

There are many other herbs that may be used to treat a particular condition or a symptom of that condition. Consult an herbal guide (see Resource Guide, chapter 11) for more information about herbs that are not detailed in this chapter.

Atherosclerosis: Herbs (oral): Bamboo, garlic, hawthorn berry, lime blossom, yarrow. *Aromatherapy:* Juniper oil for massage, or rosemary oil if nerve problems as well as CAD.

The following conditions, which often accompany atherosclerosis, can also be treated with herbs.

Angina: Herbs (oral): Garlic, hawthorn berry, lime blossom, motherwort. *Aromatherapy:* Camphor oil (only 1 drop mixed with carrier oil) for massage of chest and back.

Tachycardia or palpitations: Herbs (oral): Broom, bugleweed, motherwort, passion flower, valerian. *Aromatherapy:* Lavender, melissa or ylang-ylang for massage or in a bath.

High cholesterol: Herbs (oral): Onion, garlic, ginger.

Prevention of clots (blood thinners): Herbs (oral): Onion, garlic, ginger. *Does not replace anticoagulant therapy.*

Congestive heart failure: Herbs (oral): Broom, bugleweed, figwort, hawthorn, dandelion leaf, parsley root.

The following conditions, which often accompany angina, can also be treated with herbs:

Edema: Herbs (oral): Broom, dandelion, lily of the valley, yarrow.

Hypertension (high blood pressure): Herbs (oral): Hawthorn berry, onion, buckwheat, cramp bark, garlic, lime blossom, yarrow. *Aromatherapy:* Mixture of hyssop, lavender, marjoram, and melissa to inhale or for massage.

Hypotension (low blood pressure): Herbs (oral): Broom, gentian, ginseng, hawthorn berry, kola, oats, skullcap, wormwood.

Poor circulation: Herbs (oral): Broom, buckwheat, cayenne, dandelion, ginger, hawthorn berry, horse chestnut, lime blossom, yarrow.

The following conditions, which often accompany poor circulation, can also be treated with herbs:

Local swelling of ankles or legs: Herbs (oral): Dandelion, yarrow.

Phlebitis (blood clot in leg): Herbs (oral): Arnica, comfrey, hawthorn berry, marigold externally as compress or poultice. *Aromatherapy:* Juniper or rosemary as massage oil or in a bath.

Stress: Herbs (oral): Balm, hops, lime blossom, motherwort, pasque flower, skullcap, valerian. *Aromatherapy:* Clary sage, frankincense, geranium, lavender, neroli, or ylang-ylang to inhale or for massage.

The Herbal Road to Wellness

The subtle and many-faceted herbs described in this chapter have been used successfully as cardiac remedies for centuries. Their actions are different from those of the drugs derived from them, because they support and restore all systems that contribute to heart problems as well as working on the specific problem. They must be carefully dosed (just like drugs) and used appropriately if you are mixing them with conventional medicine—do this *only* with the support and approval of your primary-care physician. When you're considering a holistic approach to heart disease, herbal medicine stands out as a strikingly efficient means of therapy.

CHAPTER SEVEN

What Homeopathy Can Do for Your Heart

Homeopathy is a method of holistic treatment formulated by an eighteenth-century physician named Samuel Hahnemann, who decided that there was more to disease and wellness than the presence or absence of symptoms. The word *homeopathy* comes from the Greek *homoion* (''similar'') and *pathein* (''disease or suffering'').

Hahnemann's principle of the ''law of similars'' stated that a small dose of something that upsets the body can act as a trigger to help heal it. This idea is in direct contrast to *allopathic* medicine, which supposes that a drug that acts in opposition to the disease *(allos* means ''different'' in Greek) can remove or suppress symptoms.

For example, a cardiologist will prescribe nitroglycerin to alleviate your angina. And yet, according to homeopathy, the pain you feel in your chest is beneficial because it is a warning sign of something more significant going on in the body. By prescribing the remedy *Latrodectus mactans* to act on the angina, he would enable the body to rally its immune defenses and start the healing process by itself. Homeopathy rebalances you in a fundamental way, and works on the whole *being,* not just the whole body.

The basis of homeopathic thought is that a person's symptom represents his own personal way of fighting a disease. By taking a remedy that corresponds to his unique set of reactions (physical, mental, and spiritual), he is pushed a little farther in the same direction. This way he is stimulated to reorganize himself around a higher state of health.

An important part of the homeopathic philosophy is that the personality of the patient helps to determine the remedy. This means that there are mental and emotional components to the remedies. An excitable, irritable type of person will probably need a different remedy than what a quiet, laid-back person would take, even if they have the same basic symptom, such as heart palpitations or chest pains.

Homeopathy, like Chinese and Indian medicine, is based on the restoration, rebalancing, and conservation of energies in the body and mind. Energy exists, just as matter does, although it is harder to track. (One type of proof is Kirlian photography, which allows us to see auras, or fields of energy around individuals.) Even if we cannot explain how the *energy* of a crude substance can heal just as effectively as the substance itself, we can certainly understand that returning the body to wellness involves a lot more than simply eliminating a set of symptoms.

How the Remedies Work

The homeopathic practitioner uses hundreds of different remedies, some of which pertain to the patient's personality, some to his emotional reaction to a physical symptom, and some to the symptom itself. The remedies are derived from plants, flowers, animals, and minerals—some are completely benign and others have a deadly origin—bee sting and snake venom, for example.

In order to make a homeopathic remedy, these crude substances are ground and mixed with water or alcohol, then allowed to steep for two weeks and filtered into a "mother tincture." This tincture is shaken briskly, a process known as *succussing,* and then further diluted to make the various potencies. Thus begins a lengthy process known as *potentiating,* or building up the strength of the remedy by breaking down the active substance with an inert substance.

Homeopathic remedies are not intended to be antibacterial or antiviral. Rather they work on the body as a whole and strengthen one's ability to resist disease and infection. They appear to have no side effects and can be used in conjunction with most allopathic medications.

How Allopathic and Homeopathic Remedies Can Work Together

Homeopaths believe in the strength of the body's "vital force," a concept similar to the Eastern idea of the qi energy that exists in every living thing. We inherit a certain energy derived from our parents as surely as we inherit our genes. This energy mixes with the energy of the earth itself and propels the mind-body throughout life. A Western medical doctor would probably concede that we each have a "will" to live, a drive that is often able to transcend disease.

So, as long as one's vital force is intact, there is no reason that homeopathic and allopathic treatment can't coexist. Immunosuppressant drugs, such as corticosteroids, would diminish the force of any homeopathic remedy. But diuretics, beta-blockers, calcium channel blockers, clot busters, and even aspirin will not interfere with the action of the remedies.

If your primary-care physician has you on these medications, and you are also seeing a homeopathic practitioner, be sure to take both forms of treatment. You should not stop taking any heart medication precipitously. If over time it's clear that your blood pressure is consistently lower, your angina is gone, and you no longer have irregular heartbeats, you can discuss with your doctor tapering off your meds slowly.

When you suppress symptoms with an allopathic drug, those symptoms often come back up again once the drug is removed. But with a holistic type of treatment such as homeopathy, the progress of healing generally moves from more vital to less vital organs. You might experience an improvement in your nervous system (less anxiety, improved mood) before getting relief of blocked circulation in your legs, for example. You also usually get better from top to bottom (your heart might show some improvement before your kidneys), and from inside out (your blood pressure would lower before the overly ruddy complexion of your face returned to normal). Your symptoms generally follow a reverse order in time too—the last symptom you got is generally the first to leave you.

Homeopathic Schools of Thought

Most homeopathic physicians are trained in more than one branch of health care. They may be licensed naturopaths, chiropractors, acupuncturists, medical doctors, or nurses. Their eclectic background enables them to draw from a range of treatment possibilities.

After doing a thorough case history that might include questions about your health history, sleeping habits, food preferences, and emotional reactions to different events, the homeopathic practitioner will prescribe a remedy he wishes you to take. You start with the remedy whose description most closely resembles your symptoms. If it doesn't work within a couple of days, the next closest remedy should be given. Sometimes a practitioner will give two complementary remedies; he or she might give *Aconite* pellets to take care of the terror of a heart attack victim while rubbing *Arnica* on the patient's chest to relieve the physical injury. By using these two complementary remedies together, the homeopathic doctor is trying to sound a chord rather than just one note in the treatment.

In addition, your homeopathic practitioner might also prescribe supplements, diet, and exercise and might suggest altering your sleeping habits. As your symptoms decreased and general health improved, he or she would taper the dosages of your remedies and possibly discontinue the remedy altogether.

There are a variety of homeopathic schools. Some believe in giving one single high dosage of a remedy and watching a patient's progress over time. But most practitioners are of the "low-potency repeat" school, and in fact most of the remedies you can buy commercially in a health food store go no higher than a 30C potency. The benefit of this type of practice is that if you've selected the wrong remedy, you can quickly reorient the body toward a different one.

The homeopathic prescriber seeks to match your symptoms with the range of symptoms listed in homeopathic guides, the repertoire of physical and emotional ingredients that describes how you feel. This means that in order to diagnose properly and get just the right remedy, it's important to look not only at the symptom itself (such as high blood pressure), but at the conditions that raise the pressure higher, such as activity, food or drink, anger or frustration. You also have to look at the situations that lower blood pressure, such as touching a pet or listening to music. When the symptom occurs, you can more easily choose the right remedy by understanding factors that affect that symptom.

Because a remedy is never given to effect a "cure," there are also different ways in which the remedies work.

Constitutional Remedies

These remedies are defined by the four basic body types. You might take a constitutional remedy for a period of months to balance your system in addition to the specific remedies you take for heart disease.

- *Calcarea carbonica* is the remedy of choice for the endomorph—a hardworking, heavyset individual.
- *Sulphur* fits perfectly with the balanced medium build of the mesomorph.
- *Phosphorus* is the constitutional remedy for the thin, wiry ectomorph.
- *Calcarea fluorica* is the remedy used most for the "dismorph," the blend of several constitutions.

Fundamental Remedies

Your personality determines your fundamental type. In addition to the specific remedies you take for heart disease, you might take one of the fundamental remedies for a period of months to harmonize the various elements of your personality. There are dozens of fundamental remedies, among which are, for example,

- *Nux vomica*—the classic type A personality, thin, nervous, and irritable, a workaholic
- *Pulsatilla*—the timid, affectionate woman who cries easily and is terribly stressed (a type E)

Lesional Remedies

These relate to a specific problem. There are dozens of these, but some examples are the following:

- *Arnica* can be used by anyone for a soft-tissue injury
- *Hypericum* can be used by anyone with injuries to the nerves
- *Calendula* can be used by anyone for cuts

If, however, the constitutional, fundamental, and lesional remedies happen to coincide, you can get really dramatic results with homeopathic treatment. By doing this you can heal on many levels at one time.

Dosage and Potencies

In the early days, as homeopathy was evolving as an art, certain individuals called provers tried out the remedies on themselves in order to set standards for a healthful dosage and to find out how much would be necessary to create disease or discomfort where none existed before. If you give a remedy to someone who has no symptoms, eventually you will "prove" that remedy in the body—that is, he or she will develop the symptom picture. Though large doses of the remedies would greatly aggravate symptoms, smaller ones would stimulate the body to act and eventually heal itself of those symptoms. The smaller the amount of the original substance, the higher the potency. The more the substance has been potentiated, the greater the healing effect.

The potency of each remedy is designated by an *X,* a *C,* or an *M* (which indicates the mother tincture diluted by ten, one hundred, or one thousand, respectively). This means that a 1X remedy is one part solution to nine parts inert substance—either water or water with alcohol; a 1C or 2X remedy is one part solution to ninety-nine parts inert (or two parts of a 10 percent solution to nine parts inert). Most homeopaths counsel you to take lower dosages, such as 6X or 12X, once or twice an hour, and higher dosages, such as 30X, only once or twice a day.

As you reach higher potencies, your remedy is greatly diluted. When you fine-tune dosages to a 12X (or 6C remedy), you have only one part pure substance diluted a trillion times! Though in a 24X potency there is no longer any amount of active substance left, what remains is the energy vibration of the remedy, and this can resonate with that of the patient, stimulating his or her own natural healing force.

When you take a remedy, you are presenting your body-mind with a "phantom" of what's wrong with you. The remedy offers your body a specific direction along which it can structure its energies for optimal healing.

Choosing the Remedy That's Right for You

In order to choose an appropriate remedy for your condition, review the general listing below and choose the remedy that corresponds most closely with your symptoms and feelings.

The remedy should be taken until it removes the first level of your problem (the pain of the angina, for example). As one layer of dysfunction clears out, you will probably need a new remedy appropriate for the next level. If you stay with the first remedy longer than you should, you'll start to have new symptoms. Certain remedies can't follow one another— they are said to be inimical because they have opposing actions. (See the individual homeopathic listings to be sure you are taking remedies in an order that is compatible.)

• Begin with the remedy that most closely matches your symptom picture.

- Start by taking two doses in the correct time period, following the instructions on the bottle or tube. For an acute problem you can take 2 or 3 of the larger pellets (#35), or one third of a tube of the micropellets (#20), or 2 to 3 drops of tincture every 10 minutes to 1 hour. (See listings on pages 144–154 for the appropriate potency. If no potency is suggested, it is safe to use either 6C, 12C, or 30C potencies.)
- Pour the pellets into the bottle cap and transfer them directly to your mouth. Place under the tongue and allow to dissolve. Touching the pellets with your fingers may alter the effect of the remedy.
- Don't allow homeopathic remedies to pass through a metal detector—this will deactivate them.
- Stop taking a remedy if you feel much better or if your symptoms persist unchanged (in which case you need a different remedy).
- Avoid ingesting anything else—foods, liquids, or medicines—for fifteen minutes before and after taking any remedy. Also, don't brush your teeth with toothpaste. Some homeopathic physicians feel that caffeine deactivates remedies and should be avoided; others say that it has no effect at all. Consult your homeopathic practitioner about caffeine.
- Never expose remedies to high heats (don't take them with a cup of hot tea, for example), or strong aromas such as mint, eucalyptus, or camphor.
- If the remedy is making a difference, continue it until the symptom is no longer apparent. If you find no relief from your symptoms, this is not the appropriate medication for your condition. Examine yourself carefully, check the list again, and select a different remedy.
- If you still find no relief, consult with a homeopathic practitioner for further direction.

How to Start a Homeopathic Treatment Program

Although it's best to have a consultation with a licensed homeopath (see chapter 11, Resource Guide, if you are looking for a referral), it is possible to treat yourself. You may purchase homeopathic remedies at most health food stores, and you can order them by mail from several reputable companies (see chapter 11, Resource Guide). **However, it is important to remember that if you have been diagnosed with heart disease, or any other specific medical condition, you should check with your treating physician before taking any homeopathic remedy.**

Homeopathy won't just remove your symptom (such as angina); it will make a global difference in your life. Perhaps, as the remedy takes effect, you'll wake up in the morning feeling that you've slept really well and have better energy and appetite. Maybe if you were drawn to high-fat, high-sugar foods before, you'll have a tendency to select a better diet and start working on your exercise and stress management regimens.

If you chose your remedy correctly, you'll start to see a difference in general health within a couple of days. If the remedy doesn't act, it's as if you haven't taken it at all, and you need to select another.

Homeopathic Remedies Frequently Used for Heart Disease

Aconitum Napellus (Monkshood)

Aconite can alleviate any type of fright or anxiety affecting the mind or body. The individual will experience tension throughout the system—and tension frequently brings on other symptoms.

Aconite does nothing to produce changes in the tissues; it has a very brief action that lasts only long enough to remove the fear. So if you are having a heart attack, and you are calling 911 or are on your way to the emergency room, and feel panicky, use Aconite to calm the fear at once. DO NOT ATTEMPT TO SUBSTITUTE ACONITE FOR EMERGENCY CARE. YOU MUST GET MEDICAL HELP IMMEDIATELY.

General indications: Patient is physically and mentally restless, feels fearful and anxious. He may feel suddenly weak and have acute sensations of burning inside.

Symptoms of heart disease: Tachycardia, pain in the left shoulder, palpitation with anxiety and fainting, tingling in fingers; pulse full, hard, tense, and bounding. You can feel the temporal and carotid arteries when sitting down.

Problem improves with open air.

Problem worse with touch; at night in warm room; lying on affected side; with music; from cigarette smoke; or from dry, cold winds.

Complementary remedies: Coffea, sulphur.

Dose: 1X to 3X for congestive conditions, but much higher dosages (50M) can be used for intense problems.

Apis Mellifica (Honey Bee)

Apis acts on the cellular tissues, causing swelling of the skin and mucous membranes. For this reason any heart problem in which the body tends to accumulate fluid can be alleviated by this remedy. Other characteristic symptoms include tearfulness, soreness, and intolerance to heat or the slightest touch.

There is no interference with medications such as diuretics.

General indications: Burning, stinging pain; puffiness; red, rosy hue; aggravation from heat.

Symptoms of heart disease: Edema and swelling; sensation of constriction.

Problem improves with uncovering, open air, cold bath.

Problem worse with touch, sleep, heat, late afternoon.

Complementary remedies: Natrum mur.

Dose: Tincture to 30C potency.

Arnica (Leopard's Bane)

Arnica, which affects the venous system, is one of the most widely used remedies for any physical trauma—it's employed similarly to an allopathic drug simply to alleviate pain. During or right after a heart attack, **for which you must seek emergency medical care,** you might rub Arnica gel on your chest or take 30C potency pellets or both. There is no interference with medications such as nitroglycerin or clot busters.

General indications: Patient has a sore, lame, bruised feeling, doesn't want to be touched; he may have experienced traumatic injuries such as falls, blows, or contusions. Arnica is useful in postoperative patients for pain and to promote healing.

Symptoms of heart attack: Severe squeezing, crushing chest pain, with or without radiation down one arm—usually the left—or into the jaw. A sense of "stitches" in the heart; pulse feeble and irregular.

Problem improves with lying down, keeping head lower than feet.

Problem worse with damp cold, movement, touch.

Complementary remedies: Aconite, Ipecac.

Dose: 3C to 30C potency. The tincture or gel can be used locally but never when there are abrasions or cuts on the skin.

Aurum Metallicum (Metallic Gold)

Aurum is the first remedy we think of for a very depressed patient, someone who feels no connection to life. It is also useful for any deterioration of body fluids and alterations in the tissues. The remedy directs itself to the blood, glands, and bone. Symptoms you might have that would indicate a need for aurum would be palpitations and congestion, arteriosclerosis, and high blood pressure.

General indications: Depression, oversensitivity, pain in head, manic-depression, spiritual inclination.

Symptoms of heart disease: Missed beats immediately followed by big rebound, palpitations; pulse rapid, feeble, irregular; hypertension; endocarditis; pericarditis; valvular lesions; feeling that the heart is enclosed in armor.

Problem worse in cold weather; from sunset to sunrise.

Problem improves with warm weather.

Dose: 3C to 30C potency. Higher potency especially for hypertension and valvular disease.

Aurum Muriaticum

This remedy may be used instead of Metallicum when the main heart problem is palpitations and angina.

Cactus Grandiflorus (Night-Blooming Cereus)

Cactus acts on circular muscle fibers and is therefore useful anytime there is a feeling of constriction—like that of an iron band around the heart. The whole body sometimes feels caged, with each wire being twisted tighter.

General indications: Melancholy and sad; constriction; pulseless, panting, and prostrated.

Symptoms of heart disease: Disturbance of blood flow, endocarditis, cardiac valve disease (particularly mitral valve insufficiency); arteriosclerosis; violent palpitation (worse lying on left side); angina with suffocation; cold sweat; iron-band feeling; pain in apex, shooting down left arm; pulse feeble, irregular, quick; low blood pressure.

Problem worse about noon, lying on left side, walking, going upstairs.

Problem improves in open air.

Dose: Tincture (best made from flowers) to 3X potency. Tinctures should be taken orally as drops, 5 drops three times daily.

Lachesis (Bushmaster or Surucucu Venom)

Lachesis is the diluted form of the poison of a bushmaster or surucucu snake. Like all snake poisons, Lachesis thins out the blood, making it more fluid—if you think about traditional Western medicine, this is what's desired in a medication such as heparin or even aspirin. As the blood stays thinner, there is less likelihood of clots forming that might block off an artery and cause a heart attack or stroke. The negative side of Lachesis is that taking too much might initiate profuse bleeding. Lachesis is a remedy that seeks an outlet—either loquacious talking, profuse bleeding or discharge, or passionate emotional outbursts. The Lachesis patient may suffer from trembling, confusion, or delirium. Lachesis is important for women going through menopause.

General indications: Waves of pain, sensitive abdomen and liver, vertigo, chronic sore throat, patient sleeps into an aggravation (wakes angrily or confused from naps); may be wide awake in the evening; symptoms are left-sided.

Symptoms of heart disease: Palpitations, hypertension, fainting spells, cyanosis (blue, bloated face) in cardiac failure, feeling of constriction with a lot of anxiety, irregular heartbeats.

Problem worse after sleep, on the left side, in the spring, after a warm bath, with pressure or constriction, from hot drinks.

Problem improves with flowing of some discharge (a period, for example, or a sinus discharge), warm applications.

Complementary remedies: Crotalus cascavella; lycopodium.

Dose: 8X to 200X potency. Doses should not be repeated frequently—if possible, take a single dose.

Latrodectus Mactans (Spider Bite)

The action of this drug is very similar to that of angina pectoris. It can be used for constriction of the chest muscles, radiating to the shoulders and back. This remedy influences the nerves and muscles and is useful during spasms, high anxiety, and weakness or paralysis of limbs. It can be employed instead of nitroglycerin for a heart attack or severe angina.

General indications: Restless and uneasy, constipated, patient wants to be on his own, away from work or social commitments.

Symptoms of heart disease: Violent pain in the center of the chest extending down arm to fingers, numbness of extremities; pulse feeble and rapid; cramping pain from abdomen to chest. Skin cold as marble.

Problem worse/improves: No specific indications.

Dose: 6C potency.

Lycopodium Clavatum (Club Moss)

This remedy is useful for ailments that gradually weaken the system and may also relate to evidence of urinary, digestive, or liver disturbance. (Congestive heart failure, diabetes, and kidney disease may affect one individual, since one system breaking down can affect another.)

General indications: Lack of discipline, inferiority, fear of commitment, flatulence, depression, irritability, right-sided ailments, afraid to be alone.

Symptoms of heart disease: Poor circulation, cold extremities, patient is thin and withered, lacks vital heat. Pains come and go suddenly. May have aortic disease, palpitations at night.

Problem worse on right side, from right to left, from above downward, from four to eight P.M., from hot or warm applications (although warm drinks are all right).

Problem improves with motion, after midnight, from warm food and drink, from being uncovered.

Complementary remedies: Calcarea, Sulphur, Pulsatilla, Lachesis, Natrum mur.

Dosage: Lower and higher potencies have equally good results. Can use 6C to 200C potencies in not-too-frequent doses.

Natrum Muriaticum (Sodium Chloride)

This remedy is the first one considered for anyone with high blood pressure since it has to do with salt consumption and fluid retention in the body. The person who has edema (swollen tissues), gout, or hyperthyroidism is a good candidate for natrum mur. This is a serious-looking person, a perfectionist.

General indications: Deep grief and sorrow, weak and weary, dry mucous membranes, coldness, wants to be alone to cry.

Symptoms of heart disease: High blood pressure, quickened heartbeat, sensation of cold around heart; fluttering, intermittent pulse that makes body shake.

Problem improves with open air, cold baths, skipping regular meals, pressure on back.

Problem worse with heat, midmorning, at seashore, lying down or talking, consolation.

Complementary remedies: Apis; Bryonia, Sepia.

Dose: 12C to 30C in infrequent dosages. Higher potencies are more effective.

Nux Vomica (Poison Nut)

This is the remedy for the classic type A personality who drives himself or herself hard and expects a lot from others. Nux is known as a "polycrest" remedy—suitable for many ailments—because most of its symptoms mimic those of the most common diseases. The Nux vomica individual tends to indulge in alcohol, tobacco, late hours, and rich food.

General indications: Oversensitive to light, noise, odors; competitive; irritable; faultfinding; impatient; chilly.

Symptoms of heart disease: Faintness, convulsions, cerebral accidents (stroke), angina pectoris, palpitations from coffee or excitement.

Problem improves in evening; with a nap or rest; in damp, wet weather.

Problem worse in morning; after eating; in cold, dry weather; with mental exertion.

Complementary remedies: Sulphur, Sepia.

Dose: 1X to 30C. Acts best when given in the evening.

Following are other, less frequently used remedies for cardiovascular problems. Some of these are fundamental remedies (relating to personality) and some will deal with conditions or feelings that might appear in a person with cardiovascular or other symptoms. Dosages of 6C, 12C, or 30C are recommended, unless your homeopathic practitioner suggests a different dosage.

Belladonna (Deadly Nightshade)

General symptoms: Sudden onset, restless, thirstless, delirium with fever, throbbing pain, flushed face. Palpitation, heart seems too large. This might be used instead of Aconite for an immediate, acute problem; however, it is not for hypertension or heart attack. Belladonna is for right-sided ailments, lacking the anxiety and restlessness of Aconite.

Problem improves with semierect posture.

Problem worse in afternoon and after midnight; with noise; upon lying down; with touch.

Bryonia (Wild Hops)

General symptoms: Very irritable, dry mucous membranes; constipation, bursting pain, thirsty.

Problem improves when lying on painful side; with rest, pressure, cold.

Problem worse with motion, touch, warmth, eating.

Calcarea Carbonica (Calcium Carbonate)

General symptoms: Forgetful, apprehensive, very sensitive to cold.

Problem improves with dry weather.

Problem worse with cold, mental or physical exertion, standing.

Phosphorus

General symptoms: Fearful, anxious; sensitive to environment such as light, noise, odors, thunder; thirst for cold water, sudden onset of symptoms.

Problem improves with sleep, cold, cold food, open air.

Problem worse with evening, touch, warm food or drink, lying on left or painful side, physical or mental exertion.

Pulsatilla (Windflower)

General symptoms: Emotional, weepy, likes attention, thirstless, needs open air, changeable.

Problem improves with open air, cold food and drink.

Problem worse with heat, rich fatty foods, evening.

Sepia

General symptoms: Indifference, sadness, chilly, anxious, depressed, indifferent to loved ones or work.

Problem improves with exercise, warm bed, after sleep.

Problem worse in morning and evening, in cold air or dampness.

Treatment by Condition or Symptom

Below is a listing of possible symptoms you may have, with appropriate remedies to try. Although only a few basic remedies are described in this chapter, there are many more possibilities, some of which are listed here. If you wish to explore them, see chapter 11, Resource Guide, for a listing of the prominent homeopathic "repertories" you can consult.

Atherosclerosis

Angina: Aconite, Arnica, Apis, Aurum, Cactus, Lachesis, Latrodectus mactans.

Anxiety (with pain in heart): Aconite, Cactus, Kali bichromicum.

Boring or bursting pain: Aurum.

Burning pain: Arnica, Aurum, Carbo vegetabilis, Hypericum perfoliatum.

Heart attack: Aconite, Apis, Arnica, Cactus, Lachesis, Latrodectus mactans.

Squeezing sensation: Aconite, Cactus, Lachesis.

Sharp pain: Lachesis, Naja, Sulphur.

Tightness around heart: Apis, Arnica, Arsenicum, Cactus, Aconite.

Palpitations: Aurum, Natrum mur, Phosphorus, Naja, Aurum, Sulphur.

Palpitations on exertion: Arnica, Arsenicum, Cactus, Lachesis, Naja, Natrum mur.

Congestive heart failure: Aconite, Apis, Glonoine, Hypericum perfoliatum, Lachesis, Pulsatilla, Sulphur.

Edema: Apis, Arsenicum, Aurum, Crataegus, Lachesis, Lycopodium.

Feeling of congestion or fullness around heart: Aurum, Lachesis, Sulphur, Pulsatilla.

Feeling weak and lethargic: Crataegus, Naja, Nux vomica.

Swelling: Lachesis, Sulphur.

Endocarditis (inflammation of the lining of the heart): Aconite, Arsenicum, Aurum, Bryonia, Cactus.

Hypertension: Natrum mur, Aconite, Crataegus, Lachesis, Veratrum album.

Pericarditis (inflammation of the membranous sac that encloses the heart): Aconite, Apis, Arsenicum, Aurum, Belladonna, Bryonia, Sulphur, Mercury.

Valve problems

Fluttering: Aconite, Naja, Natrum mur, Cactus, Nux vomica.

Murmurs: Cactus, Naja, Rhus toxicodendron.

Regurgitation (blood flows backward through valves): Cactus.

You may also wish to try one of the "polycrest remedies," which are suitable for many different problems, regardless of your personality, body type, or particular form of discomfort. These remedies cover both fundamental and constitutional problems. For heart disease, the polycrests to try are Arsenicum, Lachesis, Lycopodium, Nux vomica, Sepia, Pulsatilla, and Sulphur.

The Homeopathic Road to Wellness

The first principle of homeopathy is that our natural state is a healthy one and that we have the ability to return to it if we have strayed off the path to a disease state. Using the information provided here, you can improve the condition of your heart and help to rebalance its energies.

CHAPTER EIGHT

What Chinese and Ayurvedic Medicine Can Do for Your Heart

The traditional Chinese medical tradition and the Indian Ayurvedic medical tradition date back at least four thousand years. Both Chinese and Ayurvedic practice are based on the belief that knowledge of our minds and bodies gives us the potential to balance our systems and enhance our spectrum of wellness.

In this chapter, we'll explore the basic precepts of both types of medicine and tell you how to find a practitioner. Although you can treat yourself with herbs, nutrition, and exercise, you will need a trained physician to guide your therapy for heart disease.

Both Chinese and Ayurvedic medicine involve sensible preventive care (diet, exercise, and good attitude) and lengthy diagnostic techniques far different from anything we know in the West. Chinese medicine treats illness with herbs, acupuncture and *qi gong* (a type of breathing and exercise); and Ayurvedic medicine treats illness with herbs, healing sounds, meditation, aromatherapy, and music therapy.

Most Western physicians claim that modern medical science has perhaps 50 percent of the "answers" for disease and trauma. It is equally true that Chinese and Ayurvedic medicine have about half the "answers." So perhaps the ideal would be to combine the high-tech knowledge of the West with the ancient, tried-and-true medicine of the East, just as it's done in Japan and China today. Fully 83 percent of Western-trained cardiologists in Japan now routinely prescribe herbs within the scope of their treatment, and many will use herbal medicine before they'll ever try pharmaceutical medications, which may have deleterious side effects.

How to Start a Program of Chinese or Ayurvedic Medicine

If you're interested in pursuing either form of Eastern medicine, you will have to choose either a traditional Chinese or an Ayurvedic doctor (usually an M.D. or an N.D.) as your primary-care physician. Although you may experiment with herbal supplementation and the allied therapies discussed in this chapter on your own, if you have been diagnosed with heart disease, you will have to be under a doctor's care in order to benefit from Eastern medical practices.

The best course of action is to get a referral from someone you know; you may also consult holistic care centers in your area to find a doctor. See chapter 11, Resource Guide, for the names of professional groups that may be able to help you.

Many American hospitals currently have staff who practice acupuncture for pain reduction and drug rehabilitation. You may be able to get a referral to a Chinese doctor from a Western physician who practices acupuncture.

If you live in a community where there is a large Chinese or Indian population, it will be far easier to find a physician. Ask at the local community center or even a local health care or social services agency.

In a bonding of East and West, patients are afforded the widest option of care. Using these venerable traditions in conjunction with modern Western science, we may unravel many of the secrets of heart disease.

Chinese Medicine: The Marriage of *Yin* and *Yang*

The Yellow Emperor, Huang Ti, who reputedly lived from 2697 to 2597 B.C., is credited as the originator of Chinese medicine. His official text, *The Yellow Emperor's Book of Internal Medicine (Nei Ching Su Wen)*, which was compiled by his followers around 1,000 B.C., sets down principles and guidelines not just for the practice of medicine but for the practice of life as well. In the fifth century (around the time that Galen was a doctor in the West), the physician Chang Chung-ching detailed the uses of acupuncture, moxibustion (in which herbs are heated on the skin, see page 164), respiratory therapy, physiotherapy, and massage.

These works are based on the philosophy of Taoism (see page 90 for a discussion), which states that everything in the universe is divided into the two complementary camps of yin and yang. The first is yielding and receptive; the second, strong and untiring. These two elements of life are not opposites, according to Taoism, but rather are flip sides of the same coin. (The clearest example is water: A river is yang when it moves and flows powerfully over rocks, but it turns yin as it freezes in winter and becomes ice.) If we move in harmony with the Tao (roughly translated as ''the Way''), we are healthy; if we become out of sync with it, we may develop illnesses.

The flow of the body's energy is determined by the confluence of yin and yang in the particular organs and tissues, and on the balance of the five elements: Wood, Fire, Earth, Metal, and Water. The heart is a Fire element and a yin organ;

however, it has yang aspects as well as influences from the other four elements.

Traditional Chinese medicine is not concerned with treating the heart per se, since the organ we know of as the heart is simply part of the "viscera," which maintain the functions of storage, heating, digestion, elimination, and qi (energy) production. The heart cannot be examined as an isolated organ, but only as a piece of one continually changing organism.

Chinese Diagnosis

A traditional Chinese physician uses four diagnostic techniques. The Eastern method of looking for "clues" to an illness is far more detailed than anything you've probably encountered in your allopathic physician's office.

The four aspects of diagnosis are:

Looking

This involves attentive examination of the patient's general appearance, physical shape, manner (which involves personality), and behavior. It also involves an awareness of the patient's *jing* (the essence that guides development and reproduction) and *shen* (spirit), which our doctors might describe as that sparkle in the eye in a healthy person—or the dullness in the eye of a sick person. The shen gives vitality to the jing and qi in an individual.

During this exam, the doctor also looks at facial color to see the state of the body's qi and blood (our doctors would talk about a sallow or pale complexion in a sick person). The most important part of looking, however, is the examination of the tongue. Chinese physicians will examine the tongue's color and texture, the "mossiness" on top, and the presence or absence of bumps as well as the shape of the tongue (a "thin" tongue might result from being chilled for a long time; a "thick" tongue might come about as a result of a stomach disorder). Finally, the doctor will look at bodily secretions and ask about the patient's excretions—these include phlegm, vomit, urine, and stool.

Listening and Smelling

The doctor listens to your voice to hear whether it's hoarse or clear, weak, or strong. He'll of course listen to your breathing and coughing. The detection of certain odors is a subtle art—Chinese physicians are able to smell a "rancid" or "fishy" or "bleachlike" odor in sick individuals.

Asking

Just as any Western doctor would do, a Chinese physician takes a thorough history. In addition he'll ask questions about your body temperature, headaches or dizziness, perspiration, thirst and appetite, sleep patterns, gynecological and urological concerns, as well as the type of pain you might be feeling. The doctor will ask emotional as well as physical questions of the patient. "Are you quick to anger?" or "Are you often disturbed by nightmares?" might be two typical questions asked of a person that we in the West might designate as a type A.

Touching

The fourth exam is considered the most important because it involves taking your pulses. A good Chinese doctor is an expert at this art—not reading just one pulse but twenty-eight. In the West a pulse is used as the detector of your heart rate and rhythm; but in the East the feeling of pulses serves several diagnostic purposes, cluing the physician in to the regulation of blood, qi, shen, and jing throughout the body.

The doctor uses the index finger, middle finger, and ring finger in order to feel nine separate pulses at the radial artery at each wrist. A normal rhythm is between 4 and 5 beats per complete breathing cycle (one inspiration and one exhalation), which equals about 70 or 75 beats a minute. Chinese medicine declares that a "normal" pulse varies according to the age, sex, build, and level of fitness—an athlete has a slow pulse, a child has a fast one, a woman's is usually softer and quicker than a man's, an obese person has a slow, deep pulse, and a skinny person has a superficial one. The quality of any healthy pulse should be "lively" and elastic and should have an even beat.

The touch part of the exam also involves contact with certain acupuncture points and different parts of the body that might be sensitive. The doctor is able to see whether the skin feels moist, dry, hot, or cold, and at the same time can tell whether pressure or release of pressure causes pain or relief.

The four-tiered diagnosis would reveal one of eight typical patterns of imbalance in yin and yang, cold and hot, interior and exterior, and deficiency and excess. This points up an interesting difference from Western medicine. An allopathic physician would talk about atherosclerosis, mitral valve dysfunction, or congestive heart failure as "syndromes," or a grouping of signs and symptoms that have an underlying cause. But a Chinese physician doesn't bother to pin the signs he sees to one cause—instead he recognizes a pattern and uses it as his guidebook for treatment. These eight patterns show different types of disharmonies; through the use of acupuncture, herbs, breathing (qi gong), and mental suggestions, the patient will be helped to heal.

How Chinese Medicine Explains a Heart Disorder

It is not possible to judge heart disorders without also regulating the rest of the internal organs; therefore a practitioner of traditional Chinese medicine would spend a lot of time investigating the state of the liver, spleen, and kidneys. The blood of course would be an essential factor, but so would the qi of various organs, the state of the patient's jing and shen, and the six Pernicious Influences, or external forces (wind, cold, fire, heat, dampness, dryness, and summer heat) that might have bearing on the patient's condition.

Other considerations would be the seven Emotions (joy, anger, sadness, grief, pensiveness, fear, and fright) and of course the patient's way of life, which encompasses all the preventive health concerns of Western medicine—diet, exercise, sexuality, and miscellaneous factors such as a snakebite or burn. (Chinese medicine does not specifically prohibit alcohol and tobacco; however, there is an injunction against living in disharmony with the elements. Staying up late and carousing, for example, will drain the qi from individual organs or overstimulate those organs.)

Following is a description of heart disease as viewed by traditional Chinese medicine. It is believed that problems with the heart generally have to do with the blood and the shen (spirit):

Deficient Heart Blood and Deficient Heart Yin

Symptoms: Palpitations, forgetfulness, insomnia and disturbed dreams and sleep, feeling of unease.

Pulse and tongue: Deficient Heart Blood has a pale tongue and thin pulse, which will in turn produce a pale, lusterless face, dizziness, and lethargy. Deficient Heart Yin will have a reddish tongue, rapid and thin pulse, possible night sweats, warm palms and soles, and an agitated manner.

Western analysis of the patient: Hypertension, arrhythmias, hyperthyroidism, depressive neurosis.

Deficient Heart Chi and Deficient Heart Yang

Symptoms: Lethargy, palpitations, pain in the chest, and "muddled" shen.

Pulse and tongue: Deficient Heart Chi has weak and irregular pulses that might be knotted or intermittent. Deficient Heart Yang would be the same but more severe. The tongue will be pale, swollen, and moist. An extremely sick individual may have yang so deficient that it collapses. The patient may have blue-tinged skin and be sweating and shaking with extreme cold. He may have a barely recognizable pulse and may be close to death.

Complications: The patient may also have Deficient Lung Chi because the entire chest is involved; he may also have Deficient Kidney Yang, since the kidneys are the source of yang in the body.

Western analysis of the patient: Cardiac insufficiency, atherosclerosis, angina, general weakness.

Patterns of Congealed Blood

Symptoms: Stabbing pain, purple face and tongue (yang symptoms) combined with lethargy, palpitations, and shortness of breath (yin symptoms).

Pulse and tongue: Pulse will be choppy and wiry (in between yin and yang). If there is a great deal of mucus obstructing the blood, the tongue will be thick with greasy moss.

Western analysis of the patient: Angina, pericarditis, coronary artery disease.

Complications: Insufficient Heart Chi or Heart Yang often precedes or accompanies this condition, resulting in stagnant blood, which is unable to move through the chest. A Chinese physician would have to determine whether the problem was a case of excess or deficiency of yin and yang, what aspects of heat and cold affected the case, and which other organs might be involved.

Acupuncture

Acupuncture is a yang treatment with yin effects because the needles penetrate the exterior of the body and offer benefits to the organs and tissues inside. A Chinese doctor will commonly use about five to fifteen needles of different thicknesses and lengths to stimulate a variety of points related to your condition.

The fine stainless steel needles, often used in conjunction with moxibustion (the burning of moxa—mugwort—an herb that helps with the conduit of qi), are placed at various acupoints along one of the twelve meridians of the body. The points at the outskirts of the heart meridian, for example, can be stimulated, and energy blockages removed along this pathway.

The Chinese analysis of acupuncture credits it with moving blocked energy along the meridian pathways. If there's something wrong with an organ, for example, pain in the heart, it will show up along the entire meridian. The action of the needles affects the qi and blood in the meridians and therefore affects all the organs. So acupuncture can balance yin and yang by taking away excess, increasing a deficiency, warming a cold problem or cooling a hot problem, or increasing circulation by getting a stagnant area moving again.

Western analysis of acupuncture reveals several different benefits. The first is that it apparently triggers the release of beta-endorphins in the brain (these are natural opiates that give us a sense of well-being). A second explanation for acupuncture's success is the gate theory. Needle stimulation jams the transmission of pain from the brain to an affected organ. But recent research shows that there's more going on than just pain reduction. A study in Shanghai indicated that the use of acupuncture caused an increase in the production of immune-related substances such as immunoglobulin and specific antibodies to fight disease.

STANDARD MERIDIAN ABBREVIATIONS

LU	Lung	CV	Conception Vessel
LI	Large Intestine	Ki	Kidney
SP	Spleen	Pe	Pericardium
TW	Triple Warmer	UB	Urinary Bladder
St	Stomach	GB	Gallbladder
SI	Small Intestine	Li	Liver
HT	Heart	GV	Governing Vessel

The twelve meridians take the names of eight of the body's internal organs (although Chinese medicine does not target any one organ in treatment) and four other locations:

- The Triple Warmer is the pathway linking Lungs, Spleen, Kidneys, Small Intestine, and Urinary Bladder.
- The Pericardium is the outer protective shield of the Heart. It begins in the chest, then links the Upper, Middle, and Lower parts of the Triple Warmer before descending down the center of the right arm and hand.
- the Governing Vessel runs up the spine from the coccyx, passes through the brain and comes over the top of the head, ending at the upper lip.
- The Conception Vessel runs from the perineum between the legs up the midline of the body to the lower lip.

Acupuncture in the Treatment of Angina

For centuries Chinese doctors have stimulated the point Pe6 (Pericardium 6) for relief of chest pain. Various modern case studies from a variety of countries show that many

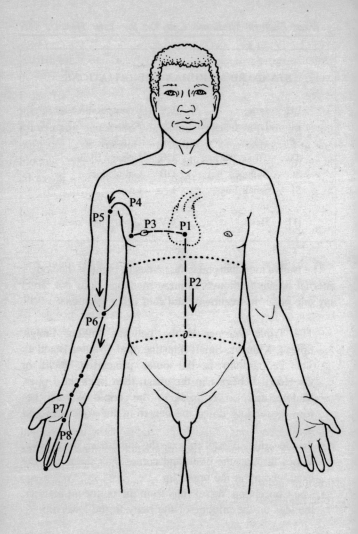

THE PERICARDIUM MERIDIAN

patients prefer acupuncture to nitroglycerine for angina because it provides long-term benefits as opposed to short-term relief.

The treatment is typically two needles applied at P6 for thirty minutes, with hand stimulation every five minutes for one to five treatments. Just this brief therapy gives most patients from two to six months of pain-free existence, without any need for medication. (Many Chinese doctors prescribe herbs to be taken in conjunction with acupuncture treatments.) The younger the patient and the shorter the history of pain, the more effective these treatments are.

The dramatic reduction of angina via acupuncture is probably due to a regulation of the two sides of the autonomic nervous system (the sympathetic and parasympathetic), which connect up to the coronary arteries via the vagus nerve. Stimulation of the P6 point in dogs shows marked increase of blood and oxygen circulation to the heart tissue—a reasonable explanation for the disappearance of angina symptoms in former sufferers. The stimulation of the needles raises the body's own defensive ability to fight cardiac injury by increasing coronary blood supply and oxygen flow.

Acupuncture appears to have startlingly good effect on many different conditions. Some studies show improvement in treating valve disease and improving the function of the left ventricle, while others indicate improvement in blood pressure and ability of the body to break down atherosclerotic plaque as well.

Acupressure Treatments for Heart Disease

If you are not under the care of a Chinese medical practitioner, you can still use finger pressure (acupressure) to get some temporary relief of various symptoms of atherosclerosis. If you seriously intend to adapt a Chinese medical

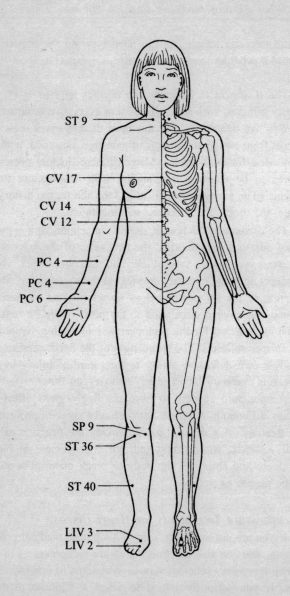

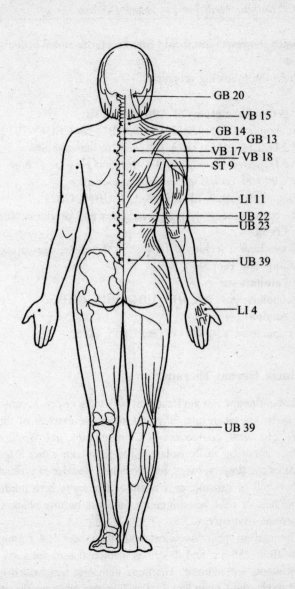

GB 20
VB 15
GB 14
GB 13
VB 17
VB 18
ST 9
LI 11
UB 22
UB 23
UB 39
LI 4
UB 39

regimen, however, you should consult a professional acupuncturist.

Press the following acupoints:

For general symptoms of Atherosclerosis:
Acupoints: UB15, UB17, UB18, UB23, St9, St36, CV12, Li2, Li3, LI4, LI11, GV13, GV14. Also massage St9.

For Hypertension (*CAUTION—If blood pressure is higher than 200/100, do not use acupuncture at all.*):
Acupoints: GB20, LI11, St36, Li3, UB15, UB22.

If you have accompanying headaches and dizziness, add Li2, GV34.

If you have a feeling of fullness in the chest, nausea and vomiting, add Pe6, St40, Sp9.

For Palpitations:
Acupoints: Pe4, Pe6, HT7, UB4, UB15, UB39.

For Angina:
Acupoints: CV14, CV17, Pe6, UB15, HT5.

Chinese Herbal Therapy

Herbal therapy is a yin treatment with yang effects because the herbs are taken internally and affect the exterior of the body. The active compounds of Chinese herbs, like Western herbs, cannot be easily isolated. You may take either a tea made of the flowers, twigs, and branches; powder of ground herb; a pill or capsule; or a tincture. The same herb might dispel heat or cold, boost immune function, remove phlegm, or restore vital energy.

The earliest pharmaceutical text, the *Shan Hai Ching,* dates from 250 B.C. and describes medicinal uses for sixty-eight plants and animals. The more complete text, which is used today, the *Chung Yao Ta Tsu Tien,* describes nearly six thousand medicinal herbs (although only three hundred are commonly used in treatment).

There are three basic types of herbs:

- Imperial Class—nontoxic and rejuvenating
- Ministerial Class—toxic or nontoxic effects promoting mental stability
- Assistant Class—toxic properties used for treatment of disease states.

Drugs created from herbs are also categorized as to

- Temperature—cold, cool, warm, or hot
- Flavor—pungent, sweet, sour, bitter, salty
- Direction—ascending, descending, floating, or sinking

A "hot" drug might restore vital (yang) energy to the body and might therefore be used in the treatment of a Deficient Heart Yang condition; a "bitter" drug might get rid of heat or dampness; a "sour-warm" combination could have astringent effects.

The toxic compounds that do exist in some Chinese herbs come in such weak concentrations that they cannot do any damage to healthy tissue, but will break down diseased tissue. All Chinese herbs (which are rarely used singly) must be used over several months or longer for any effect to take place. As you will see, there are some duplications of Western herbs, such as mint, skullcap, and foxglove.

Dosages

Dosages for Chinese herbs are completely individual and must be set for you by your Chinese medical practitioner. He or she will prescribe combinations of herbs and often give you the mixture already made. Or, if you live in a metropolitan area that has a large Chinese population, you may be sent to a Chinese pharmacy to have the mixture made for you. You may be prescribed teas to take several times a day, or pills, tablets, tinctures, or pressed juices.

- *Combined teas:* Pour boiling water over 1 to 2 teaspoons of dried herbs and allow to stand 10 to 15 minutes.
- *Tinctures:* Take 10 to 20 drops in a few tablespoons of water, three times daily, half an hour before meals.
- *Pills or tablets:* As your doctor prescribes.
- *Pressed juices:* You will need a juicer or a hand squeezer. Many of the herbs are derived from fruits, which are rich in vitamins and minerals. Take juice diluted with a few tablespoons of water, three times daily half an hour before meals.

Herbs for Hypertension

Siler and Platycodon Formula (Sang-Feng-Tung-Shen-San) is for hypertension accompanied by obesity and constipation. This combination contains Chinese angelica root, ma-huang (ephedra), cnidium, peony root, gardenia fruit, ginger rhizome, forsythia fruit, siler root, licorice root, chinchieh herb, nitrous sulfate, paichu (white atractylodes rhizome), rhubarb rhizome, field mint, platycodon (balloon flower root), skullcap root, gypsum, and talc.

Rehmannia Eight Formula is for older people with hypertension and kidney complications. This combination includes yam, cornus, hoelen, cinnamon twigs, Chinese foxglove, aconite root, and tree peony bark.

Herbs for Palpitations

Ginseng and Tang-Kuei Formula (Jen-Sheng-Tang-Shao-San) is for palpitations accompanied by cold feet, dizziness, stiff shoulders, and anemia. This combination contains Chinese angelica root (Tang-Kuei), cnidium, peony root, alisma, cinnamon twigs, paichu rhizome, hoelen, ginseng root, and licorice root.

Atractylodes and Hoelen Combination (Ling-Kuei-Chu-Kan-Tang) is for headaches, dizziness, and severe palpitations.

This combination contains hoelen, cinnamon twigs, licorice root, and paichu.

Herbs for Angina or After Heart Attack

Bupleurum and Dragon Bone Combination (Chai-Hu-Chia-Lung-Ku-Li-Tang) is for severe chest pain with difficulty breathing. This combination contains bupleurum (hare's ear root), pinellia rhizome, skullcap root, jujube fruit, gingerroot, ginseng root, cinnamon twigs, oyster shell, hoelen, rhubarb rhizome, and dragon bone.

Tonics

Radix Astragalus (*Huang qi*) is a qi tonic that tonifies the Spleen, Stomach, Qi, and Blood. It lowers blood pressure and increases endurance.

There are also blood tonics. For example, Paeoniae Alba (*Bai shao*) nourishes and stabilizes the blood and alleviates pain; it lowers blood pressure and has a mild anti-inflammatory effect. Radix Polygonum Multiflorum (*Ho shou wu, Fo-ti*) tonifies and detoxifies the Liver and Kidneys; it decreases cholesterol levels. Radix Rehmanniae (*Shu di Huang*) tonifies and stabilizes the blood and nourishes the yin organs; it lowers blood pressure and serum cholesterol.

The Medicinal Effect of Herbs and Other Growing Things

The best-known Chinese cardiovascular tonic is panax ginseng, which is a stimulant and restorative for the heart and other organs. The Chinese variety of this root contains many important vitamins, such as niacin, folic acid, B_{12}, pantothenic acid, and biotin. As a heart tonic this herb by itself (2 cups of ginseng tea daily on an empty stomach) can work wonders.

Ginseng lowered cholesterol levels in rats fed a high-cholesterol diet, although it will not alter a normal cholesterol level. The herb will also adjust blood pressure (either abnormally high or abnormally low) to a normal level but will have no effect on someone with a routine pressure. An interesting distinction between the effects of a drug and the effects of an herb are that a drug causes changes in a normal state, whereas an herb acts only when there is need—in an unbalanced or dysfunctional situation.

A Chinese fungus, a mushroom known as *ling zhi* (or *reishi* in Japanese), is also credited as an exemplary cardiovascular tonic, and either the mushroom or a tea made from it can be consumed daily with no side effects. This burnt-orange mushroom with a lotus-pad-shaped cap can lower blood pressure and calm the nervous system. It is a bitter, warm herb and alleviates symptoms such as knotted or tight chest, cold hands and feet, anxiety, and deficient Heart qi. Researchers have found that this fungus thins the blood and prevents clots, lowers serum cholesterol and triglyceride levels in the liver, and lowers blood pressure. One of its components is angiotensin-converting enzyme, which is the same as the Western cardiac drug known as an ACE inhibitor.

Qi gong

The particular Chinese breathing and exercise technique known as *qi gong* (pronounced *chi gung*), or "breathwork," attempts to move energy throughout the body from the *tan tien*, or "field of elixir," the place where that powerful elixir of air, oxygen, and energy comes from. The tan tien is a point about three inches down from your belly button and three inches inside. (Whether the actual point exists or not is not important—this is the center of your body and therefore a good point on which to orient the breath.) Clinical observations indicate an over 85 percent success rate for those who use qi gong to treat hypertension. It also reduces symptoms of coronary artery disease, affords a more regular electrocardiogram, and offers better cardiac function.

How does breathing accomplish all this? Technically, of course, what you're doing when you breathe is affording better oxygenation to the blood—thus solving one of the primary problems of cardiac dysfunction. The *Yellow Emperor's Canon of Internal Medicine* describes it this way: "One must breathe in the essence of life, regulate one's respiration to preserve one's spirit and keep the muscles relaxed." *Dō-In,* an ancient form of exercise dating back to the few first hundred years B.C. in the Han Dynasty, combined regulated breathing with physical movements and was used in therapy for treating a variety of ailments. Today there are special clinics, sanatoriums, and hospitals in China to treat chronic disease with qi gong.

Although there are many different types of qi gong, all require the patient to do something active in order to take care of the disorder, which may result from a deficiency *(xu),* an excess *(shi),* or cold or heat. In learning the correct breathing technique and exercises for your heart condition, you must be able to regulate the mind, the respiration, and the appropriate body position.

Focus Attention on the Source of Your Breath

Start by concentrating on your tan tien. Inhale and exhale, using the image of this point to draw the breath in and out. Think about the energy that accompanies the breath as filling your body and being stored there. As you exhale, eliminate the carbon dioxide and some oxygen, but remain filled with qi.

Use Your Mind to Move Your Breath

It's not enough to breathe in and out; you have to send your mind to the same place the breath is going. So if your aim is to lower your blood pressure, you must visualize the blood coursing through your system and consciously relax the blood as it travels from your head to your neck, to shoulders, arms, wrists and hands, back, chest, waist, abdomen, and finally your legs, calves, and feet.

How to Breathe

Expand your belly as you inhale and allow it to contract as you exhale. (Anyone with heart problems must use easy, natural breaths and not exert undue stress on the internal organs.)

Body Position Helps Your Qi gong

If you are in relatively good health, you can do your breathing as you sit, stand, or walk; however, if you have advanced heart disease, you should practice the breathing as you lie on a flat, well-padded surface. Place your hands at the tan tien point so that you can guide the inhalation and exhalation more efficiently.

According to Chinese medicine, qi gong helps to relieve tension in the cerebral cortex and reduces the excitability of the sympathetic nerves. The end results are a dilation of the peripheral blood vessels, lowering of blood pressure, and a slower pulse.

There is also indication that qi gong can help improve hemodynamic reactions, promote circulation in the coronary arteries, and improve myocardial metabolism.

Ayurvedic Medicine

The meaning of Ayurveda, translated from the Sanskrit, is *Ayus,* "life," and *Veda,* "knowledge" or "science." The basic principle of this science of life is avoiding disease by maintaining a balanced awareness of everything in our lives.

Each person's road to wellness and path back from illness is unique to him or her—yet each of us has the capacity to heal ourselves with diet, exercise, herbal therapy, meditation, and adjunct practices such as aromatherapy (breathing in the essence of healing plants), primordial sounds, music therapy, and several other practices.

The diagnostic techniques of Ayurveda bear some resemblance to those of Chinese medicine—the taking of multiple pulses, for example, and pressure-point stimulation (*marma* therapy, done with finger pressure instead of needles). The most striking difference from Chinese medicine is the Ayurvedic belief that treatment is based on one of three body and personality types.

Ayurveda charges us to stay well—it's an obligation we owe to everyone on the planet. One of the Vedic verses reads "It is our duty to the rest of mankind to be perfectly healthy, because we are ripples in the ocean of consciousness, and when we are sick, even a little, we disrupt the cosmic harmony." The implication is that we are one with every other human, plant, and animal that has ever lived or will live. Healing the heart, then, is quite a responsibility!

If you are switching over from Western allopathic care to Eastern medicine, you must bring all your medical records from your former physician, copies of your EKG and echocardiogram, if any, and all the prescriptions you may have for your heart condition. Your Eastern doctor will want to wean you slowly from these medications.

Using the *Doshas* for Self-Diagnosis

Ayurvedic medicine is grounded in a belief in certain personal types, which make up your "nature" or *prakriti.* The division into types is dependent on your build, personality, behavior, moods, tastes, and talents. You may be one of three *doshas,* or functions of the mind-body system. Everyone contains a bit of each dosha within himself or herself, but we have tendencies that place us more in one category than another.

Vata dosha controls movement. Vata individuals tend to be thin and wiry, always on the go, quick learners, often anxious, often cold.

Pitta dosha controls metabolism. Pitta individuals are of medium build, usually high intellect, with a strong digestion and sharp hunger and thirst. They are good speakers and tend to be fair-skinned. They may be aggressive and quick to anger.

Kapha dosha controls structure. Kapha individuals tend to be relaxed and slow but powerfully built, with great physical strength and endurance—although they have a tendency to put on weight. They sleep heavily and have a slow digestion. They are slow to learn, but once they do, they remember.

You may be a combination of two doshas or even rather balanced among all three, but you'll be prescribed different herbs, sounds, diet, exercise, and lifestyle suggestions, according to the influence of your dosha or doshas.

The Cardiac Predispositions of the Doshas

Each dosha is associated with an organ system.

Vata imbalances have to do with movement, which means that a Vata might just as easily have very good or very poor blood circulation. Vata is also allied with the nervous system and its connections along nerve pathways to the muscles and blood vessels. Typical Vata heart problems are hypertension, valve disorders, arrhythmias, or arterial spasms.

Pitta is responsible for metabolism and also regulates the heat of the body. Part of its function is to balance blood chemistry, but it also has the job of keeping the heart contented. A person whose heart is out of balance might suffer emotionally, but might also have a heart attack. Because Pitta imbalances tend to be hot and sharp, a typical Pitta heart problem would be angina and possibly myocardial infarction.

Kapha is responsible for structure and moistness. This means that Kapha imbalances of the heart might lead to chest congestion and excess fluid around the heart. If you are a pure Kapha, you will be predisposed to have a high cholesterol level and/or congestive heart failure, possibly complicated by obesity or diabetes.

Symptoms and Conditions of Your Dosha

Once you have consulted with an Ayurvedic physician, you will understand your dosha's own predilection for imbalance. You and your doctor can then treat what's wrong before it becomes a chronic condition.

Vata imbalances are associated with pain, spasms, cramps, chills, or shakiness.

Pitta imbalances are associated with inflammation, fever, heartburn, or excessive hunger or thirst.

Kapha imbalances are associated with congestion, fluid retention, lethargy, and mucus discharge.

A simple imbalance may be located in one dosha; however, a chronic condition such as heart disease means that all the doshas are out of balance. For example if you are a Vata type and under undue stress, your blood pressure may rise (Vata is involved). But if this condition continues without treatment, you may start to have angina or arterial spasms (Pitta is involved). And you may start to feel terrible fatigue and lethargy as you get sicker (Kapha is involved).

The goal of Ayurvedic medicine will be to rebalance the doshas and restore you to health.

Balancing the Doshas

Health requires order. If your natural constitution has a balance of Vata 3, Pitta 2, and Kapha 1, it should remain that way. If you were to come down with the flu and were filled with mucus, your Kapha moving up to 4 and your Pitta down to 1, as long as you came back into balance when the flu was over, you'd be fine. It's when the disorder remains and the doshas are in a continual state of imbalance that the disease process moves into the deeper tissues and structures of the body. Since the different doshas have different requirements, the treatment will depend on your particular type. However, all types will be directed to make some changes in diet, exercise, daily routine, and seasonal routine.

In addition to a prescribed diet and activity schedule for your type, you would be instructed to meditate daily. According to Deepak Chopra, M.D., who has popularized the use of Ayurvedic medicine in this country, "physical impurities in cells have their equivalents in the mind . . . as damaging to us as any chemical toxin." (Read chapter 4 to learn how to meditate.)

Your physician will counsel you to do the following in order to balance your dosha:

Balancing Vata requires

Quiet/meditation	Staying warm
Drinking fluids	Stress reduction
Rest	Regular habits and meals
Sesame oil massage	Ten P.M. bedtime
Low-impact exercise	

Balancing Pitta requires

Moderation in everything

Balance of rest and activity

Exposure to natural beauty

Laxative foods

Enemas

Moderate sports (hiking, biking)

Staying cool

Taking leisure time

Avoidance of caffeine, tobacco, alcohol (stimulants)

Avoidance of hot, spicy foods

Balancing Kapha requires

Stimulation

Weight-control program

Avoidance of sweets

Clear sinuses with saltwater rinse

Regular, vigorous exercise

Staying warm and dry

Variety of experiences

Dry massage (done with raw-silk gloves)

Panchakarma: Purification of the Body

There are five steps to ridding the body of impurities:

1. Oleation, or the ingesting of clarified butter for several mornings in a row to minimize digestive action.
2. Laxatives, to flush out intestinal impurities.
3. Oil massage using an oil specified for your body type. This is a full-body massage intended to direct the toxins to move toward the eliminative organs. A related treatment, *shirodhara,* involves a drip of warm oil on the forehead to relax the nervous system.
4. Sweating, to open the pores and flush impurities through the sweat glands.

5. Enema, to cleanse the intestinal tract. There are about one hundred medicated enemas used in Ayurveda.

Primordial Sounds

The idea of meditating, or clearing the mind in order to heal the body, leads naturally to the use of mental powers more refined than thinking. This type of therapy delves into the faint vibrations we can pick up as we become more skilled at silencing the busy whir of thoughts and feelings inside. It is believed in Ayurveda that when we are out of balance, certain of our vibrations have become distorted; however, we can restore them to normal if we develop our awareness.

The sound *Om,* used by many meditators, is an example of the connection to the "harmony of the spheres," described by many philosophers. This sound can be chanted or heard silently. The primordial sounds are far more subtle than this, however, and must be taught to you by a qualified Ayurvedic physician. By using the sound as an organizing tool for the brain, Ayurveda states that it is possible to restructure a faulty connection, for example, between the brain and the coronary arteries when we feel the pain of an angina attack.

Aromatherapy

The power of smell (and its companion, taste) is stronger than we think, because of its location in the brain. Whereas the other senses are centered in the cerebrum (the cognitive center), smell and taste reside deep in the middle of the brain in the limbic system. This emotional center also houses the master gland of the body, the hypothalamus. When we are aware of an odor, our nasal passages detect it, then pass it on through olfactory cells in the nervous system to the hypothalamus. This gland not only communicates via hormonal production with all the other glands, but on its own it is responsible for regulating many bodily functions, including temperature, thirst, hunger, sexual arousal, blood sugar levels, and growth. It is also close to the tiny hippocampus, which controls memory.

You can see, then, how significant smells can be because of the brain receptors that pick them up. A whiff of a particular spice or herb can alter physiological responses because of the proximity to this influential brain center. And our memories of times when we were healthier and stronger can actually influence our ability to become healthier and stronger.

The mind can take in literally thousands of smells. Your Ayurvedic physician will have to prescribe the particular aroma you need for your heart condition. (This "prescription" will depend on your dosha(s) as well as the dosha that is out of balance. There will be specific aromas used for your particular imbalance that has led to the symptoms of angina, atherosclerosis, valve disorder, arrhythmias, congestive heart failure, or recovery from heart attack or bypass surgery.)

The Ayurvedic aromatic oils are sold in health food stores and holistic centers, and you can mail-order them from a variety of sources (see Resource Guide, chapter 11).

Balancing Vata requires a mixture of warm, sweet, and sour aromas, such as basil, orange, rose geranium, and clove.

Balancing Pitta requires a mixture of sweet and cool aromas, such as sandalwood, rose, mint, cinnamon, and jasmine.

Balancing Kapha requires a mixture of warm aromas with spicy overtones, such as juniper, eucalyptus, camphor, clove, and marjoram.

How to Make an Aromatic Oil Elixir

Place 10 drops of oil in a teacup to warm over a hot plate, and sit nearby. You may read or meditate, or you can set up an aromatherapy infuser before bed and sleep while you inhale the scent.

Repertoire of Herbs for Ayurvedic Healing

The Ayurvedic repertoire of herbs is enormous, and the whole plant is always used in treatment. Ayurveda feels that the strong chemical action of one compound will be offset by others in the plant. Like foods, herbs are classified according to the six tastes—sweet, sour, salty, bitter, astringent, and pungent. Herbs, however, are more specific in their actions than foods.

As in Chinese medicine, an Ayurvedic physician always starts with a "tonifying" mix, to support and nourish the body, whether it is simply run-down or whether the patient is suffering from a specific illness, such as heart disease.

To support Vata, take gotu kola and ginseng.

To support Pitta, take aloe, comfrey root, and saffron.

To support Kapha, take elecampane and honey (used as an herb in therapy).

Some of the herbs prescribed for heart disease are the same as in Western herbal medicine; others are only available in Indian markets (if you live in a neighborhood that has one), or directly from your Ayurvedic physician. See chapter 11 for addresses of mail-order supply companies.

General-wellness herbs are available in health food stores or Indian markets; however, specific herbal formulas for heart disease must be prescribed and dosed by your Ayurvedic doctor. They will be determined according to your dosha and will be given to you by your medical practitioner, or you will be told what to order through mail-order companies and Ayurvedic organizations (see chapter 11, Resource Guide).

Herbs for Ayurvedic Healing

Cayenne *(Capsicum annum)*

To correct: Insufficient Kapha and Vata; excess Pitta.

Properties: Stimulating, sweat-inducing, regulates blood flow.

Symptoms: Poor circulation, chronic chill.

Preparation: Infusion or powder mixed in water or food.

CAUTION: Do not use if you have ulcers, gastritis, or any inflammation of the gastrointestinal tract.

Chamomile *(Anthemis nobilis)*

To correct: Insufficient Kapha and Pitta; excess Vata.

Properties: Sweat-inducing, antispasmodic, analgesic, calming.

Symptoms: Headaches, stress, indigestion.

Preparation: Infusion (hot or cold) or powder mixed in water or food, paste.

CAUTION: Large doses may induce vomiting.

Goldenseal *(Hydrastis canadensis)*

To correct: Insufficient Kapha and Pitta; excess Vata.

Properties: Bitter tonic, antibiotic, antibacterial, antiseptic, laxative.

Symptoms/conditions: Diabetes, obesity, swollen glands, and lymphatics.

Preparation: Decoction or powder mixed in water or food; paste used externally only.

CAUTION: NEVER use more than 3 grams a day—overuse may cause vertigo, emaciation, debility.

Hawthorn Berry *(Crataegus oxycanthia)*

To correct: Excess Pitta and Kapha; insufficient Vata.

Properties: Stimulant, vasodilator, antispasmodic, diuretic.

Symptoms/conditions: Atherosclerosis, hypertension, blood clots, high cholesterol, heart weakness/palpitations.

Preparation: Decoction or powder mixed in water or food.

CAUTION: Overuse may cause ulcers or colitis.

Bala, Indian Country Mallow *(Sida cordifolia)*

A species in the mallow family (which is related to the cotton root plant), Bala is an effective cardiac tonic and stimulant. It is nourishing to the nervous system and is nutritive to the entire body. It also promotes tissue healing.

To correct: Insufficient Kapha, Pitta, Vata.

Properties: Tonic, rejuvenative, diuretic, stimulant, aphrodisiac, calmant.

Symptoms/conditions: Heart disease, convalescence.

Preparation: Decoction, decoction in milk, powder mixed in water or food, paste, medicated oil.

Lotus *(Nelumbo nucifera)*

Lotus seeds and lotus root act as a tonic for the whole body, the seeds being more specifically a cardiac tonic. They can be ground up and eaten (5 grams three times daily) with rice.

To correct: Insufficient *Pitta* and *Vata;* excess *Kapha.*

Properties: Nutritive tonic, rejuvenative, aphrodisiac, calming, regulates blood flow.

Symptoms/conditions: Heart weakness, bleeding disorders.

Preparation: Decoction or powder mixed in water or food, or the root and seeds.

CAUTION: Overuse may cause indigestion or constipation.

Reaping the Benefits of Chinese and Ayurvedic Medicine

Both traditional Chinese and Ayurvedic medicine have withstood the test of time—probably millions of people over the centuries achieved excellent results from both of these healing arts. Once you've found a practitioner you trust, you can assimilate into Eastern culture—at least medically—for the better health of your heart.

When you are learning more about your options for health care, you may find that your thirst for knowledge opens up new possibilities, and that you discover some therapies that are not commonly recognized or appreciated. In the following chapter, we'll discuss biofeedback, chelation, Reiki, reflexology, and environmental change.

CHAPTER NINE

Other Complementary Treatments for Heart Disease

In the wide lexicon of therapies that complement traditional allopathic care, several stand out. Although not as widely known or commonly practiced as nutrition and supplementation, herbal medicine, homeopathy, and stress reduction, the therapeutic techniques we'll cover in this chapter are often used in conjunction with others to give a wider range of care.

Biofeedback, chelation, Reiki, reflexology, and environmental change have their staunch advocates and critics—and there are pros and cons to each type of treatment.

Biofeedback

Biofeedback uses electrical instruments to teach self-awareness and help you alter body processes you formerly thought of as involuntary. If you choose biofeedback therapy, you will be hooked up with sensors to a machine that gives a readout on a variety of body functions, such as heart rate, blood pressure, and temperature. As you watch the lights or hear the sounds that correspond to activities of your nervous and endocrine systems, you *relearn* how your body can respond under stress.

You are taught to monitor your body, get feedback from the mechanical helper beside you, and use it to change the way your body reacts. After a few sessions on the machine, most individuals are able to perceive what the body is doing without mechanical help and to alter its functions.

Through training you can be taught easily, for example, to avoid the triggers that might raise your blood pressure. If you think angry thoughts, your heart will race and you will push the pressure up. You will be able to see those indications on your readout and understand that you must use your voluntary state of consciousness to alter your involuntary responses. Calming your mind, using relaxation techniques such as meditation and visualization, actually thinking your blood pressure moving down as though it were descending an escalator, you can change the readout.

How the Biofeedback Machine Works

The biofeedback machine serves as an intermediary between the person and his environment. Since stress is our *perception* of a particular event or feeling, this is one way to alter our unconscious reaction to fear or anxiety. By concentrating on the output of the machine, you switch your focus from external (the event) to internal (how the event made your body react).

The machine and the person connected to it form a closed loop where information can be processed. The person receives messages from the environment and reacts in a particular way, which registers on the screen. He is then able to alter the output of his involuntary systems by exerting conscious control. This is a three-phase process.

THE PHYSIOLOGICAL PHASE

The body releases energy (either physical, chemical, thermal, or electrical) and the machine measures it. When you are stressed and your heart races and palms sweat, you produce chemicals that carry an electrical charge that may result in cell movement (muscles tensing) or cellular secretion (output of stress hormones, gastric acids, etc.). This biological activity also throws off heat. The machine can register all of these various reactions.

THE PSYCHOPHYSIOLOGICAL PHASE

Mind and body link up to coordinate the energy-releasing systems (nervous and endocrine systems). The nervous system is composed of two parts: the involuntary (autonomic) system and the voluntary system. And the autonomic system is again divided into the *sympathetic* nervous system, which is responsible for the "fight or flight" response—heart speeding up, stomach churning, pupils dilating, muscles tensing—and the *parasympathetic* nervous system, which brings us back to stasis by instituting a calming effect.

The goal in biofeedback is to circumnavigate the instinctive sympathetic response and go directly to the voluntary system.

THE LEARNING PHASE

As the machine provides you with information about the performance of your central nervous system, you are increasingly able to exert voluntary control on body systems. By receiving the feedback from the machine, you can recall a similar event that stressed you and use problem-solving techniques to wind up with a different result.

Using the Process to Reduce Heart Disease

Since the cardiovascular system is very responsive to stress, biofeedback is a particularly effective tool to help heal the heart.

The chief influences on heart rate are muscle activity (such as exercise and hard physical labor), infection, and emotion. If you are aerobically stimulated, all you have to do to get your heart rate back to normal is to slow your body down. The better your muscle tone, the faster you'll return to normal. If you're sick, you have to attend to the symptoms that made you ill before you can get your heart rate back to normal. But emotions are something we can control. And biofeedback machines can help us to do this.

The measurement of cardiac activity gives a clear picture of the balance between the sympathetic and the parasympathetic nervous systems. Heart rate changes occur during the anticipation of an event as the nervous system gets ready for a response from the muscles. If you're upset, your heart races, you may have palpitations, and your arteries constrict, which raises blood pressure. But if you learn to calm yourself and consciously think, "Slow down," and see your heart rate decline on the screen in front of you, you can use that experience the next time you feel stress in order to get your body back in balance.

The Benefits of Biofeedback

When you use biofeedback, you are reinforcing a new memory of how your body feels when you react with relaxation rather than stress. One of the best biofeedback tools to increase elasticity in the arteries is the galvanic skin response meter, which allows control over dilating and constricting blood vessels. A band is attached to one of your fingers, which is linked by an electrical wire to the machine. The temperature of your finger is registered on the machine's readout.

Blood vessel constriction is governed by the sympathetic system (which reduces blood flow to the fingers); dilation is governed by the parasympathetic system (which increases blood flow as we relax). We tend to get cold, clammy hands when we're stressed and warmer hands when we feel comfortable. If your thermal sensor shows low temperature when you feel nervous, you can think, "My hands feel heavy and warm. . . . I am quiet and peaceful . . . I feel warm and relaxed," and try to increase peripheral blood flow in your fingertips.

The Drawbacks of Biofeedback

If we can practice changing heart rate, blood pressure, and vessel elasticity, it would appear that we could conquer heart disease. But is that true?

Unfortunately the heart and mind are exceptionally complex mechanisms, and it's not always clear that by circumventing a dangerous health problem we are healing it. We may just be taking it in a different direction. In an experiment with rats, the animals were paralyzed with a drug and monitored for vascular activity in the ear. The group that learned to relax (dilate) the vessels in one ear more than the other received a pleasurable electrical stimulation. The clever rats learned how to do this trick by figuring out how to slow their heart rates. The less clever rats increased their heart rate. It would appear that figuring out how to relax would make us healthy, if not wealthy and wise. But these small biofeedback experts who slowed their hearts uniformly died of heart failure or other cardiac disease. The mechanical performance of altering heart rate is only one aspect of what's going on— there are hundreds of biochemical changes that occur in a reversal of the stress response, just as there are in the activation of a stress response. Perhaps *too* much control is just as bad as not enough.

It is still uncertain as to whether biofeedback will make a

significant difference in changing the course of heart disease. However, the *awareness* it offers of our bodily functions is well worth the experience.

How to Find a Biofeedback Practitioner

If you are interested in biofeedback, you will need to consult a professional first. After you have used the machines at a biofeedback center for approximately ten sessions, you will be able to continue your practice at home, either with a small machine or instrument you can purchase or without mechanical assistance. Consult the Resource Guide, chapter 11, for the number of the national organization, where you can be referred to a practitioner in your area. Many hospitals and holistic centers also have biofeedback treatment programs.

Chelation Therapy

Chelation therapy involves the intravenous infusion of a prescription medicine into your bloodstream in order to clean plaque from arteries and restore blood flow. It appears to be a chemical substitute for bypass surgery, and because it is noninvasive, it is far less traumatic to the body and mind. There is still considerable debate as to whether it works as well as surgery or can maintain good health for as long a period of time.

The chemical process involved in this therapy is quite simple: The medicine used in the infusion forms an amino acid ring around target metals that build up in the body, and the metals then bind to the ring. As the medicine is washed out of the body through the kidneys, the metals are washed out with it. Basically this is the same process used in detergents in order to scrub rings from bathtubs or float dirt out of your laundry.

Chelation comes from the Greek word meaning "claw." The medicine—a combination of EDTA, vitamin C, magnesium, B vitamins, and several different minerals—grabs on to a metal like a claw and doesn't let go until it's out of the body.

The Blood-Cleaning Chemical, EDTA

EDTA (ethylenediaminetetraacetic acid) is a chemical that leaches metals from the body, thereby cleansing it of free radicals that damage cell membranes. This in turn improves calcium and cholesterol metabolism and stops the buildup of new plaque on the arteries. EDTA removes poisons—lead, mercury, aluminum, and cadmium—that interfere with proper cell function. By taking abnormal calcium deposits out of the blood cells and the muscle layer of arterial walls, it helps to restore smoothness to the vessel walls.

Once the metallic elements are washed from the cell, the plaques can shrink down so that blood flows more freely. Cleansing the walls of the cell of this debris also makes them more elastic and flexible. Since healthful chemicals also bond to EDTA (zinc, vitamin B_6, and other vitamins), these are restored to the body either orally, intravenously, or intramuscularly at the end of the chelation therapy.

The Future of Chelation in Heart Disease Treatment

Chelation therapy is still very controversial, and most conventional physicians are not in favor of it because they feel that although it has been sufficiently tested under rigorous scientific controls for other conditions, it is not as certain how chelation affects the heart and circulatory system. Although the FDA approved this treatment as a method of treating lead poisoning and several other conditions in the early 1950s, they have not approved chelation for heart disease.

However, lead levels have been found to be higher in hypertensive individuals and may be one cause of kidney disease in some patients with high blood pressure. Lead, which becomes more toxic when left in the body for long periods of time, is one of the metals that seem to bond best with EDTA. An article in the *New England Journal of Medicine* reported that chelation therapy may be highly effective in the treatment of hypertension.

Individuals who have completed treatment report that they have less leg and heart pain when they exercise and that their memory, hearing, eyesight, and sense of smell are improved. They also report that they no longer experience skipped heartbeats, extra beats, or rapid beats and that their heart rhythms appear to be regular.

The side effects of this therapy, if any, may include irritation of the veins, fever, headache, and fatigue. Usually these symptoms vanish after your physician has adjusted the dosage of the medication in the infusion or the frequency of your treatments.

This therapy can safely be used simultaneously with medications such as beta-blockers, calcium channel blockers, and blood thinners such as heparin.

How to Find a Chelation Therapist

There are approximately four hundred physicians in the United States today who perform chelation therapy. Holistic physicians and naturopathic doctors are the most likely medical practitioners to be trained in chelation therapy.

The physician you consult for this treatment will use it as part of a broad-based heart-healthy program that will include nutrition and exercise, smoking-cessation, and vitamin and mineral supplementation.

During the treatment you sit in a chair, where a very slow intravenous drip of the medication mixed with vitamins and minerals is introduced into your system. Most individuals need twenty to forty sessions, each lasting about four hours. The total cost may be from two to four thousand dollars.

If you wish to find a therapist in your area, you can contact the American College for Advancement in Medicine (ACAM), 1-800-532-3688, for a referral.

Energetic Therapies: Reflexology and Reiki

The Western medical tradition and many of the therapies covered in this book approach the body from a biological and chemical perspective. However, in the East, and in other therapies, the body is seen as an energy source, and illness as blocked energy. When the energy is free flowing, the body becomes better able to help itself heal—this is the goal of both reflexology and Reiki.

Reflexology

Foot reflexology is the practice of massaging and stimulating specific areas of the foot that correspond to other parts of the body. By working on the foot, you are improving general circulation and facilitating healing.

The treatment originated in the early 1900s when a doctor named William Fitzgerald observed that pressure on one area of the body could produce an analgesic effect elsewhere. Other practitioners who studied Fitzgerald's work decided that the human form can be charted as a map, divided into ten equal longitudinal zones running the length of the body, from the top of the head to the tips of the toes.

When you coordinate the location of the internal organs along the paths of the ten zones, they correspond to the fingers and toes. Each finger and toe falls into one zone, and any organ lying along that path can be manipulated through the finger or toe (the feet are generally considered a better conduit for releasing congestion and tension than the hands). Direct pressure applied to any part of a zone affects the entire zone in the same way that stimulating an acupoint on a particular meridian affects all the points along that meridian. This means that working on the whole foot will relax and release the whole body.

How Reflexology Can Assist in the Treatment of Heart Disease

When you touch the bumps and planes of the feet, you may be able to detect problems elsewhere. For example, if you are having a mild attack of angina, you may wish to alleviate as much of the pain yourself as you can by using reflexology so that you can be coherent enough to speak with your doctor on the phone. By locating the referral area along the appropriate zone on your foot and working it with your fingers, you may be able to dull the pain in the heart area so that you can get a full breath.

Why does this work? An attack of angina or palpitations brings on a powerful stress reaction, and an outpouring of the "fight or flight" hormones keeps the panic and pain high.

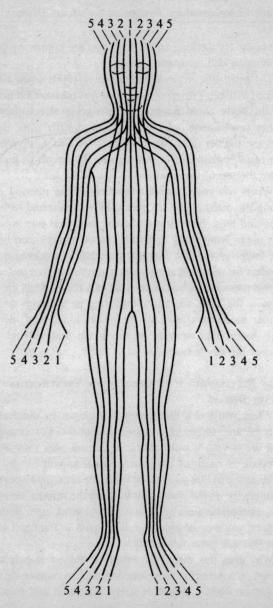

THE TEN MERIDIANS

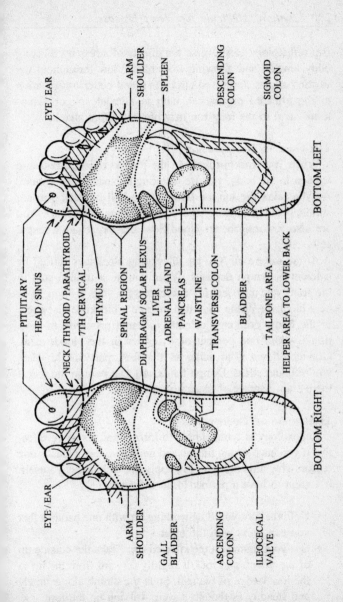

PITUITARY
HEAD / SINUS
NECK / THYROID / PARATHYROID
7TH CERVICAL
THYMUS
SPINAL REGION
DIAPHRAGM / SOLAR PLEXUS
LIVER
ADRENAL GLAND
PANCREAS
WAISTLINE
TRANSVERSE COLON
BLADDER
TAILBONE AREA
HELPER AREA TO LOWER BACK

EYE / EAR
ARM
SHOULDER
SPLEEN
DESCENDING COLON
SIGMOID COLON

BOTTOM LEFT

EYE / EAR
ARM
SHOULDER
GALL BLADDER
ASCENDING COLON
ILEOCECAL VALVE

BOTTOM RIGHT

But reflexology can reverse the effects of stress by relaxing body tension and allowing freer blood flow throughout the various organs. Improved circulation and better oxygenation to the afflicted organs can help to alleviate major symptoms—and in the long run may prevent future attacks.

THE GOAL OF REFLEXOLOGY

When you work on areas in the foot to relieve stress and tension in the body, you are restoring balance to the system. As you relax the toe, or areas on the ball or heel, you are simultaneously relaxing the corresponding body part. You are also restoring better blood flow and oxygenation to the cells.

At the same time you are alleviating blockages caused by calcium or lymph deposits. When you hit a trouble spot in the foot, you may feel a "crunchiness"—this is thought to be a blockage in the zone that mirrors a blockage elsewhere in the body. Although calcium is found primarily in bone tissue, about one percent of it resides in the bloodstream. Gravity allows it to settle in the feet, particularly when you're under stress. Lymph fluids, too, can pool in the feet if there's an increase of tension in that zone.

TECHNIQUES OF TREATMENT

Reflexology is quite simple to learn—but it's more effective if you have strong fingers and good leverage. (This is one reason why, although you can apply the techniques yourself, it's great to have a partner to do it for you.)

- Hold the foot you'll be working on with one hand so that you can press with the other.
- Use your thumb on the affected area. Take the outside tip of the thumb and rock it slightly forward from the tip to the lower edge of the nail. Slide the thumb along slowly and steadily as though it were walking up the foot.

- Use the four fingers to hold the toes back and pull them forward. While you are "walking" your thumb, the fingers can play back and forth as you raise and lower your wrist. Sinking your wrist increases pressure; raising your wrist decreases it.
- In order to pinpoint a small area, you can stop your thumb walking and allow the thumb to hook into the point. Then pull back across this point with your thumb.

WORKING ON THE HEART THROUGH THE FEET

Although the corresponding area for the heart is located on the ball of the left foot between the second and third toes, you will be working on the *chest/lung* area on both feet because the heart sits in the middle of the body. This basic area should be used for all heart ailments, from atherosclerosis and angina to valve disorders, congestive heart failure, edema, and arrhythmias.

Start with the right foot and hold the toes back with the left hand. Thumb-walk around the entire area from the base of the toes through the ball of the foot, working systematically up the four lines that match up with the spaces between the toes. Be sure to include the curved portion from the edges into the ball on both sides of the foot.

When you've completed working with one hand, balance yourself by shifting hands and repeat the process.

When you've completed the right foot, move on to the left foot and thumb-walk once with each hand. Pay particular attention to the heart location—be aware of any sensations (rapid heartbeat slowing down, irregular heart rhythm becoming regular) that occur over time as you work on your feet.

Since the "fight or flight" hormones are secreted from the *adrenal glands,* you should work on them next. Pull back your toes, and you will notice a tendon that runs the length of the foot. The spot for the adrenals is located inside this tendon, around the arch of the foot.

If you have had a heart attack, you may also work on the *sigmoid colon,* which is located on the lower left curve of the left foot, about midway between the edge of the foot and the center point. This portion of the colon often traps gas, which can put additional pressure on the rest of the body. Relieving the gas may help you breathe more freely, thus getting better oxygenation to the chest cavity.

If you have hypertension, you should work the *solar plexus, kidneys,* and *adrenals* in addition to the other points. The solar plexus area is a band that lies flat across the foot, just between the bulge of the bone beneath the big toe and the arch. The kidney area is located on each foot right at the inside top of the adrenals (just inside the arch). High blood pressure can damage the kidneys; the solar plexus is involved in the stress/alarm reaction of the body, since it is rich in nerves and muscles used in this reaction.

Reiki

Reiki, a Japanese healing art, means "universal transcendent spirit." The energy that is emanated in a Reiki treatment is part of the life-force energy that runs through all of us—the goal of this therapy is to channel it specifically for healing.

The power of touch is a long-honored method of healing. Spiritual leaders have performed "miracle cures" in line with the words and example of Jesus ("If you lay hands on the sick, they will be healed"), and there are many practitioners today who claim to be able to alleviate pain and disability through the laying on of hands. However, the Reiki touch is significantly different from spiritual-healing touch and is reputed to work in a much more effective manner. The individual who gives a Reiki treatment is known as a channel because he or she has been "tuned" to a higher vibratory level in order to draw energy from the universe and apply it in a therapeutic manner. When the channel lays hands on you, the appropriate amount of energy needed to work on whatever problem you might have is immediately drawn through the channel's body and into yours. If you are trained as a Reiki channel, you can draw this healing energy for yourself as well.

During a Reiki treatment, the one being worked on usually feels a glow of incredible warmth around the area being touched. The feeling of warmth, tingling, or pulsating generally lasts as long as the energy is emanating strongly to that area.

The person being healed is the determining factor in any treatment. You can't just sit there and be healed—rather you must concentrate on allowing the energy to reach your blockages. Reiki is said to transform not just the physical body but also the etheric body—that hard-to-describe element that many of us call spirit. According to energetic therapy, when the spirit is strong, the body can heal far more quickly. A Western doctor would probably say the immune system is responsible for healing; however, the two are not mutually exclusive. When you truly desire to receive healing energy, it is possible to change your mind-body chemistry.

THE HISTORY OF REIKI

During the mid-1800s, Dr. Mikao Usui, dean of a small university in Kyoto, went on a personal pilgrimage to discover why the powerful type of healing attributed to Buddha and Jesus was no longer being performed. The culmination of his quest was a twenty-one-day fast and meditation on top of a mountain. On his last day, he had a vision of light and energy that was so overwhelming, he began to run down the mountain. But as he ran, he tripped and cut his toe. When he reached down and grabbed it, the bleeding stopped, and the toe was completely healed.

Usui used his healing abilities far and wide, but what was different about his technique was that he insisted that the people he was healing assist in the process. They could not be passive, but had to take responsibility for their own well-being.

Reiki was brought to America by a Japanese-American woman named Hawaya Takata in 1935, and she trained others to take this talent out into the world. Currently there are approximately three hundred Reiki masters who teach this art. You can usually learn the first degree of attunement in a weekend, which will give you the tools you need to help yourself heal.

How Reiki Can Assist in the Treatment of Heart Disease

The format of a Reiki treatment concentrates first on the endocrine system. As you lay hands on the various glands of the body, you are reaching several systems at once—the energy channeled through you affects the nervous system, which triggers the production of neurotransmitters as well as glandular hormonal secretions. The endocrine system also communicates with the etheric or spiritual body, so that energy is channeled there as well.

In doing a treatment, the Reiki channel would first ascertain whether your problem was acute or chronic. If you had just experienced a heart attack, you would be in an acute state, and any treatment would bring on what's known as a healing crisis. As you received Reiki energy, your symptoms might return even more strongly than before. This would be a sign that you had reached a level of toxic buildup, which the Reiki energy would ignite, similar to the way a sudden flame burns up a match head entirely. This is what happens chemically when you get an infection—your immune system fights it and you develop fever or redness at the site. The end result, however, is enormously beneficial.

Chronic conditions, on the other hand, don't usually bring on a healing crisis. If you had had tachycardia or hypertension for several years, you would be a chronic case. Your immediate symptoms might lessen over the course of the first few sessions, and might vanish over the next few months.

The emotions may also be healed during a treatment, and various organs are related to certain symptoms. A person with angina, for example, has "heart pain" in the chest, between the ribs and inside the shoulders. The abdomen also stores a good deal of our anger, fear, love, and hate. It's a good idea, as you're being worked on, to concentrate on these emotions and feel them balance out as healing takes place.

How to Do a Reiki Treatment for Any Heart Ailment

If you decide to be trained as a first-degree Reiki channel, you will be able to work this treatment on yourself, or you can consult a Reiki channel for treatment.

The movement of energy should go from the general to the specific. This means that you (or your Reiki channel) would start by stimulating the various glands of the body and then work your way to the organs involved. Hold each position for approximately 10 minutes. You may have some signals as to when to move on—usually the heat or tingling in your hands decreases as the energy passes through that area.

- Start by placing the hands over the eyes and sinus area.
- Move to the temples, the ears, and the occipital lobe at the base of the brain.
- Leave one hand at the base of the brain, the other over the forehead, covering the hypothalamus, the pituitary, and the pineal gland.
- Move to the throat (the thyroid) and lymph glands below the jaw.

- Move to the sternum (the thymus). Spend 15 minutes here, as the thymus is the gland that produces the protective white blood cells of the immune system.
- Move to the heart and solar plexus (the adrenals). You should give extra attention to this position—remain here for 15 minutes.
- Move to the liver (below the right rib cage), the upper lungs (one hand on each lung), and the spleen-pancreas area opposite the liver.
- Move to the *hara,* or main energy point three fingers below the belly button. (This point is the same as the Chinese tan tien.)
- Move to the ovaries for women (above the pubic bone) or above the lymph nodes in the groin for men (top of each thigh).
- Move to the knees (they are said to govern our fear of change).
- Finish the front of the body at the feet.
- Then move to the back of the body, starting with the shoulders and moving slowly down to the sacrum.
- You may wish to return to the heart area at the end.

The Future of Reflexology and Reiki in Heart Disease Treatment

Both disciplines have their proponents and detractors. The proponents say that energy blockage is the chief source of all illness and that by relieving it, you can not only remove the symptoms of heart disease but actually encourage the body to heal itself. Anecdotal evidence of individuals who swear by these therapies is very strong, and there are also preliminary scientific studies that show promising results.

In an experiment at St. Vincent's Medical Center in New York, forty-six patients, some with congestive heart failure and some with other chronic illnesses, became significantly stronger after treatment. They all showed an increase in iron content of their red blood cells, and their symptoms improved or disappeared.

Detractors say that while reflexology and Reiki both *feel* good and are certainly relaxing, that's about the extent of their therapeutic value. Unfortunately, the scientific studies that have been done to date are on small numbers of individuals, and it is difficult to measure data in these elusive fields.

One thing is certain—there are no side effects or contraindications to either treatment, and they are worth exploring for their calming, holistic value if not for their actual healing benefits.

How to Start a Reflexology or Reiki Program

One session with a certified reflexologist or Reiki channel will probably cost from thirty-five to fifty dollars in most parts of the country. You can contact the Center for Reiki Training or the Reflexology Research Project (see Resource Guide, chapter 11), and you may also find practitioners through holistic health centers or the bulletin boards of health food stores and in bookstores specializing in alternative health care and spirituality. Some hospitals may offer reflexology and Reiki as part of therapeutic nursing programs, or in post–heart attack or bypass-surgery rehabilitation.

There is no formal licensing for this work. Reiki and reflexology practitioners must be certified; however, it is still up to you to determine whether the individual from whom you're receiving therapy is doing you any good.

You can become a certified Reiki channel yourself by studying with a Reiki master—there are three degrees of study, which become increasingly more expensive. After taking the first-degree program, you will be able to work on yourself.

You can become a certified reflexologist by taking a course at a holistic center or massage school. Reflexology is generally part of a larger course of study that includes anatomy, massage, tai chi, and pressure-point theories.

Environmental Change

The problems of living at the end of the twentieth century are extensive. We are all too overwhelmed, too pressured, too wrapped up in details that often obscure our perspective of the larger picture. We are stifled by pollution—the air we breathe, the noise we hear, the discarded garbage we stumble over are certainly detriments to our lifestyle. One of the major handicaps to being healthier is not just *how* we live but *where* we live. Is it possible that moving to a kinder, gentler place could heal the heart?

What About Climate and Altitude?

Balmy climates are good for those with heart problems. Too much cold can trigger an angina attack, and even walking out of a comfortable house into 20-degree weather can overstimulate the heart. Very hot weather may also contribute to the development of heart disease. A Michigan study revealed that hypertensive individuals who had succumbed to heatstroke in the past were five times more likely to develop heart disease in the future than those with no previous symptoms.

A study done by the National Institutes of Health on thirty-two metropolitan areas showed that deaths from heart disease were consistently lowest when the air temperature was in the sixties and seventies. This also means that during especially blistering days, you should stay indoors in the air-conditioning.

Although extremes of temperature can shock the heart, the same is not true of altitude, unless you're talking about moving to the Alps. It would appear that the air is uncomfortably thin for those with cardiac problems at about 14,000 feet; however, there is no appreciable difference between living at altitudes of 5,000 and 10,000 feet.

Country Versus City Living

The old story about the country mouse and the city mouse proves a point: If you are a person who thrives on the stressful challenge of an urban setting, you will languish in the country. And if you feel terrible anxiety away from your beloved trees and babbling brooks, you will be miserable in the city. Either condition could prove damaging to your heart.

If you have no preferences at all, or have lived happily in both locations, then country or even suburban life is probably more calming than any city existence, and therefore is better for anyone with heart disease. The American Lung Association reports that deaths from coronary heart disease are 37 percent higher for men and 46 percent higher for women in cities.

The most significant biochemical factor that argues in favor of a healthier lifestyle, of course, is the air pollution of most cities. Carbon monoxide is the culprit.

This noxious gas takes the place of the oxygen the body needs. Even in those with no symptoms of heart disease, exposure to daily city air may bring on upsets in cardiac rhythm. Carbon monoxide affects cardiac function in five ways:

- It aggravates angina after more than 90 minutes' exposure.
- It aggravates spasms of the arteries after 2 hours.
- It can change electrocardiogram readings, even in normal healthy individuals after 4 hours of exposure.
- In healthy individuals, it can produce the same or similar symptoms of heart disease as smoking.
- In patients who have suffered heart attacks, it can lower their chances for survival.

Although it may not be practical for you to consider moving right now, it's worthwhile when you're thinking about adopting a healthier lifestyle. And of course the younger you are and the sooner you get out of the bad air and into the good, the faster you'll feel better. But it is never too late to make any decision that will contribute to better heart health.

When you're thinking city versus country, there's another factor to take into consideration. In cities, people live closer together, and they lack not only psychological but physical space to reduce their stress. The classic experiment where rats are forced to live nearly on top of one another in overcrowded cages proves the point. When rats have no room to lie down and have to fight to hold on to each scrap of food, they are more likely to develop physical and mental illnesses and to shorten their expected life span.

Having the Option to Make the Right Choice

Obviously we have more going for us than rats do, and yet the goal is still "a room of one's own." Whether it's where to live or how to open new doors with new therapies, the choice has to remain in our hands. The various therapies mentioned in this chapter can do a lot to amplify your overall health. And so can feeling with all your heart—which we'll discuss next.

CHAPTER TEN

Love and Affection
and Your Heart's Well-being

The heart has long been thought of as the seat of the emotions. We say that we feel our heart goes out to someone when we experience love or compassion for that person. We also say that our heart can break after some traumatic event, such as a divorce or the death of a loved one.

Can you heal your heart by loving more fully? It sounds far-fetched, yet there is extraordinary evidence of couples' longevity far exceeding that of single people—precisely because they had each other to care for and be cared for.

Dr. Alexander Lowen, the founder of the therapy known as bioenergetics, goes so far as to say that the desire for erotic and emotive contact travels on the blood, and the more repressed or frustrated our feelings, the worse shape our heart will be in.

Our sexual selves also have a part to play in our heart health. Intimacy is the primary way in which we trust another enough to become completely vulnerable. As we open our hearts along with our sexuality, we can love another and ourselves as well.

So in this chapter we must explore what it really means to

love with all our heart. By understanding what it is that makes us caring, sentient people, we can set ourselves a goal of self-healing. We can learn to be kinder to ourselves, to get rid of our pain, to forgive past angers, and to renew hope, which may allow us to be healthier in the future than we have ever been.

Group Support Saves Hearts

Dr. J. J. Lynch's landmark book on isolation and heart disease, *The Broken Heart,* documents the fact that unmarried people may be at as much as five times greater risk of heart disease than married individuals. Lynch quotes studies that reveal the long-lasting effect of sorrow at the loss of love. In the six months following the death of a loved one, death rates rise sharply, and in 75 percent of the cases studied, the cause was heart disease. Very often the shock of losing somebody this close brings on sudden death, either from a massive heart attack or from an abnormal heart rhythm that careens wildly out of control.

One of the risk factors for heart disease is a lack of social support. Women statistically outlive men in this country by about six and a half years, which is a long time, living alone, to deal with poor health. And if an elderly woman has no money, she can't afford good health care and may wait too long to see a doctor when she's ailing. If she has no one depending on her and no one who really cares much whether she gets well or dies, it is difficult for her to build motivation to eat right, exercise, and change stress factors that might encourage better health.

By building a network of concerned individuals who truly care about one another, we are taking one significant step toward healthier hearts. Dr. Dean Ornish, whose cardiac program includes physical, mental, emotional, social, and spiritual elements, feels that building intimacy and community is an integral part of reversing heart disease. And one of the biggest problems to overcome is loneliness.

Increasingly, studies show that lonely people have lower immune system response. If we feel that there's no one to call, no one to count on, we may not be able to rally the necessary T- and B-cells that will help protect us from disease and heal us quickly when we're sick.

When you're alone, you think that you're the only person in the world ever to have had a heart attack or to be frightened about facing bypass surgery; but in a group, all your fears are acknowledged and treated seriously. The people around you shore you up when you are feeling miserable; they can also be counted on to come over with a casserole or pick up your mail if you're too sick to care for yourself. And likewise, when you are in better shape than one of your friends, you can offer assistance and feel needed. Group support can alleviate the chronic daily depression that is a result of believing there is no way out and no one to help.

If there is no ongoing group for heart attack or bypass survivors at your local hospital, you may find one at a church or synagogue near you. You can start your own group by placing an ad in your local paper or putting up a notice on a community bulletin board.

Emotion as a Catalyst for Better Heart Health

If you don't feel anything, you are protected from the slings and arrows of the world's emotional garbage. Right? Wrong.

A lack of affect, as it's called, is not so much a void as a type of avoidance. If we are never angry or passionate or sad or silly, we don't give our neuropeptides a workout by calling them into action. And if these brain hormones don't flow, we may be doing irrevocable damage to the heart.

When feelings do not flow, they create the equivalent of a

blockage in the emotional stream. If you think in terms of how Chinese and Ayurvedic medicine regard the body and mind, this type of repression is as bad as having stagnant qi.

Then there are those of us who feel but don't express it. If you have ever found yourself in a rage but unable to let go of your anger (possibly at a boss or other person in authority), you are well aware of the frustration and pent-up feelings that you hold on to.

Keeping anger in bumps your stress response up to high. Instead of being angry or depressed because of someone else's actions, you make yourself personally responsible for those damaging feelings.

Allow your heart to do what it needs to, to feel appropriate emotions that will assist in the healing process. Although "venting" is not something you may wish to do every day (this can create an unhelpful explosive hormone reaction just as repression does), you should give yourself permission to feel as much and as often as you want.

The Loving Impulse

"A prime risk factor for heart disease is lack of love—not sentimental love but sexually fulfilling love," says Dr. Alexander Lowen. Research shows that individuals with active sex lives have far healthier hearts. In one study, fully 65 percent of one hundred women hospitalized after a heart attack said that they were sexually dissatisfied or were unable to have an orgasm. This group was compared with one hundred women of similar ages who were hospitalized for other problems—only 24 percent of them had sexual difficulties.

One of the primary reasons for this startling discrepancy is that those who are fulfilled in love and sexual intimacy produce more endorphins, the neurotransmitters in the brain that give us a sense of well-being. And as we've already established, if you don't love yourself and you aren't happy with your life, your heart can't thrive. If you're constantly feeling stress in your personal life, you don't produce as many protective immune cells to ward off disease.

But there's an even more basic reason that sexual relationships help the heart. During lovemaking and orgasm, the body undergoes a physiological release. There is a rush of blood to the peripheral organs, followed by a softening and relaxing of all the tissues, including the interior of the arteries. So the better your sex life, the more vital and viable your circulatory system. While making love, you also breathe more fully and take in more air—consequently the blood that's circulating gets better oxygenation.

The flip side of love, of course, is anger. Loss of love, sexual and otherwise, can engender the production of damaging stress hormones (adrenaline, noradrenaline, and cortisol). The abrupt departure of a loved one, either through death or divorce, can often trigger a heart attack. "I felt as though my heart would break" is a refrain we hear often from those in deep mourning. Absence of love can also bring on feelings of despair, hostility, and loneliness. Psychologist Catherine Stoney of the American Psychosomatic Institute has done research indicating that angry people metabolize fats more slowly than relaxed, comfortable people and have higher cholesterol levels. So it is conceivable that years of rage can clog arteries as surely as a fat-laden diet.

When we are angry all the time and lose the capacity to love, we feel numb, stiff, and tight. And this exterior manifestation may actually be mimicking the internal tightness of the arteries and their inability to carry sufficient blood to the heart. When the coronary arteries stiffen and eventually block up, this can bring on a fatal heart attack.

Touch a Pet to Lower Blood Pressure

The best stress reliever for your heart may be your dog or cat. Your friends and family may criticize you or be unsympathetic; however, the unconditional love you receive from your pets can be an untapped source of physical benefits.

Studies in nursing homes have shown that elderly individuals who had the opportunity to hold and stroke an animal a couple of times a week saw great improvements in health. Not only was their blood pressure lowered during the time they cuddled with the pet, but it remained low for hours afterward. Their spirits were lifted by watching the antics of small puppies and kittens, and they were also able to anticipate a pleasant experience on the days when they did not come into contact with the animals.

People who have pets at home have an additional advantage of developing a relationship with that animal. It has been documented that very often a sick individual will remain functional simply because he has a pet who relies on him for food and comfort. He can't become bedridden and die, because who would take care of his cats? Even following a heart attack or bypass surgery, these individuals seem to rally back to health faster because there is some small creature dependent on them.

If you don't already own a pet, this is a good time to consider adopting one. You don't have to spend much money—a mutt or an alley cat is free except for vaccinations when you first adopt. A dog or cat may turn out to be the best doctor you ever consulted.

Laughter as a Means of Healing

Norman Cousins, the former editor of the *Saturday Evening Post* and adjunct professor at UCLA's School of Medicine, was stricken with a life-threatening disease that involved his connective tissue for which there was no known cure. Cousins decided to heal himself with a battery of Marx Brothers movies and vitamin C. He found that by clearing his mind and allowing it to focus on the silliness of the old comic routines, he was able to change his attitude about illness and death. Laughter, he found, alleviates panic; the deep belly laughs also give the body the opportunity for deep breathing we rarely get during the course of a day.

Cousins's treatment was not new, although it was not scientifically proven. In the 1950s, a Harvard psychologist named Gordon Allport had postulated that humor, like religion or climbing a mountain, gives a better perspective on your own being and how you fit into the scheme of life and society. It's been said that we laugh at someone slipping on a banana peel because the experience really could hurt and bring on tears. But stepping back and looking at the event as an omnipotent being sees it, we are able to appreciate the indignity of someone standing up and suddenly falling down because of his or her own lack of awareness.

Students at a university who were shown a short comedy film were better able to counteract the effects of stress in their lives and to think up solutions to problems. They were able to go from "functional fixedness" to "creative flexibility." Laughter is the salve on our emotional turbulence, but it also puts us in our place, giving us our comeuppance for being too intense or serious.

Prayer as a Means of Healing

A cardiologist by the name of Dr. Randolph Byrd conducted a controlled, ten-month study of 393 patients at San Francisco General Hospital and found that those who were prayed for (by home prayer groups) had marked improvements in their heart disease over those who were not prayed for.

Each patient had from five to seven people praying for him each day. The prayer groups were given the first names of their patients as well as a brief diagnosis and description of their condition. By the end of the study the group who'd received the prayers were five times less likely to require antibiotics, three times less likely to develop pulmonary edema, and none of them required endotracheal intubation (an artificial airway made in their throat). Fewer patients in this group died. Prayer apparently helped in the healing process.

But what is prayer exactly? It is certainly a part of many belief systems—one can pray to a deity, but one can also offer personal prayers for someone we love without the intervention of a divine presence. In order to explore the nature of spiritual healing, psychiatrist Dr. Daniel J. Benor made a search for various studies that showed "the intentional influence of one or more people upon another living system without utilizing known physical means of intervention." He found over a hundred experiments (mostly on laboratory animals) that indicate that ordinary human beings have the ability to trigger biological changes in other organisms.

Several of the experiments he looked at tried to inhibit the growth of fungus cultures or bacteria by the use of concentration from various distances. In one of these experiments, the subjects were able to retard growth of the fungi in 151 out of 194 culture dishes. In another, growth was inhibited in 16 out of 16 trials, even when the concentrating was done at a distance of fifteen miles away.

If it's possible to stop the growth of organisms in a petri dish, why can't we stop them from growing in an individual? Could we in fact get a friend to pray away the plaque from our arteries, or inhibit our production of stress hormones? Could we do it for ourselves?

Dr. Larry Dossey, a medical doctor who has been using prayer in his practice for years, says that either directed or nondirected prayer is effective in creating change. The practitioner can have a goal and an outcome in mind—for example a prayer can be offered to make a heart attack less severe, or to make recovery from a stroke both swift and complete so that there will be no loss of function. Or if there's no known diagnosis and you're not exactly sure how to direct the body to behave, you can also pray for "what will work best."

The power of prayer cannot be formally documented in people as it can with lower forms of life, because the human spirit is unknowable and there are so many variables when it comes to getting well or staying well.

You can use prayer in your daily life, even if you do not consider yourself a religious or observant person. Here are some suggestions:

- Settle yourself and relax thoroughly before you begin to pray. You may pray silently or aloud, using a standard written prayer or your own words.
- Organize your prayers around the belief that they serve as an additional immune boost to your system or the person for whom you are praying.
- Pray daily, both for your own good health and for another's. Select that person carefully and use good visual imagery to see his or her face and body in your mind as you concentrate on the person.
- If you are praying to heal some dysfunction or rid yourself of a symptom, do it slowly—because the healing process is a slow one. Concentrate on the whole body, mind, and spirit, not just on the affected organ or tissues.
- Pray for others' well-being in addition to your own.
- Be aware that the potential for healing through prayer is very powerful and must be treated with respect.

Love Is Strong Medicine

Caring about ourselves and others may have an untapped potential in cardiovascular therapy. Love is one vital component—perhaps the most vital—to send us in the right direction when we're healing ourselves. If we remember that holistic care aims for an enhancement of wellness rather than just an eradication of disease, we cannot help but be good to ourselves—to our hearts, our souls, and our minds.

Everything else we do—the good nutrition and supplementation, the vigorous activity, the stress management, the herbs, homeopathic remedies, Eastern medical treatments, and mind-body approaches—all complement the essential therapy. That therapy is self-love, which extends from our mind, body, and spirit outward to others. To heal the heart, we must care enough to send the very best and make sure, over a long life span, that it always reaches its destination.

CHAPTER ELEVEN

Natural Resources for Heart Disease

When you're attempting to coordinate medical and natural therapies and philosophies, you have to know just where to go for the most up-to-date, comprehensive information. Below is a listing of resources—books, organizations, and items to make life easier—that will assist you on your road to good heart health.

Insurance for Complementary Therapies

Wellness Plan
100 Foster City Boulevard
Foster City, California 94040
1-800-925-5323

The American Western Life Insurance's Wellness Plan is available to residents of California, Utah, Colorado, New Mexico, and Arizona. You must choose a primary-care physician from their network; however, you also have a choice of alternative and allopathic doctors on this plan. You must have an annual "wellness" exam and appropriate testing and are then covered for twelve visits per year to a variety of specialists, including acupuncturists, Ayurvedic doctors, hypnotherapists, and others. The plan pays for herbal and homeopathic remedies and vitamins that are prescribed for particular conditions.

Alternative Health Plan
P.O. Box 6279
Thousand Oaks, California 91359-6279
1-800-966-8467

Alternative Health Plan is available to subscribers all over the country, and there is greater freedom of choice with practitioners than in the Wellness Plan. The specialists you may see include acupuncturists, Ayurvedic doctors, homeopaths, naturopaths, chiropractors, and doctors of traditional Chinese medicine. The plan does not cover vitamins but will pay up to $500 per year for homeopathic and herbal remedies prescribed by one of their physicians. They also cover twelve sessions of bodywork when prescribed by a physician. Major medical, hospitalization, and surgery are all included.

Oxford Health Plans
800 Connecticut Avenue
Norwalk, Connecticut 06854
1-800-444-6222

Oxford Health Plans, the fastest-growing HMO in the Northeast, covers members in Connecticut, New York, New Jersey, and Pennsylvania. Oxford is currently developing a program, set to go into effect in 1996, that will offer its members the option of selecting a naturopath or homeopath as their primary-care physician.

Mutual of Omaha
Mutual of Omaha Plaza
Omaha, Nebraska 68175
(402) 342-7600

For the past three years, Mutual has covered Dr. Dean Ornish's reversal-of-heart-disease program at various demonstration sites around the country. If you are a Mutual subscriber, you can get coverage for participation in Omaha, New York City, Des Moines, Fort Lauderdale, and Columbia, South Carolina.

National Organizations

Nutrition

American Dietetic Association
216 West Jackson Boulevard, Suite 800
Chicago, Illinois 60606
(312) 899-0040

Center for Science in the Public Interest
1501 16th Street, NW
Washington, D.C. 20036
(202) 332-9110

Aromatherapy

National Association for Holistic Aromatherapy
3072 Edison Corner
Boulder, Colorado 80301
(303) 444-0533

Herbal Medicine

American Herbalists Guild
P.O. Box 1683

Soquel, California 95073
(408) 464-2441

Northeast Herbal Association
P.O. Box 146
Marshfield, Vermont 05658-0146

Homeopathy

International Foundation for Homeopathy
2366 East Lake E., No. 301
Seattle, Washington 98192
(206) 324-8230

National Center for Homeopathy
801 Fairfax Street, Suite 306
Alexandria, Virginia 22314
(703) 548-7790

Homeopathic Educational Services
1-800-359-9051 (orders)
(510) 649-0294 (information)
Will send you books, remedies, tapes, software, and
home-study courses on homeopathy.

Holistic Health Care

Center for Natural Medicine, Inc.
1330 Southeast 39th Avenue
Portland, Oregon 97214
(503) 232-1100

A consultation, research, and diagnostic center run by
naturopathic physicians offers a range of therapies from
naturopathy to chiropractic, acupuncture, homeopathic,
and botanical medicine.

Rise Institute
P.O. Box 2733
Petaluma, California 94973
(707) 765-2758

This educational organization offers courses, workshops, and seminars to help people cope with chronic disease. The physical, emotional, and spiritual approach of the healing is based on the work of Sri Eknath Easwaren, a meditation teacher who created a program of holistic healing.

American Holistic Health Association
P.O. Box 17400
Anaheim, California 92817
(714) 779-6152

This organization publishes information on holistic approaches to health care.

American Holistic Medical Association
4101 Lake Boone Trail, Suite 201
Raleigh, North Carolina 27607
(919) 787-5146

This group of physicians dedicated to holistic medical practices may offer referrals to doctors in your area who are members.

Center for Mind-Body Studies
5225 Connecticut Avenue, NW, Suite 414
Washington, D.C. 20015
(202) 966-7338

The center provides education and information for anyone wishing to explore his or her capacity for self-care and self-healing. They also sponsor self-help groups for people with chronic illness.

Mind-Body Medical Institute
Mercy Hospital and Medical Center
Stevenson Expressway at King Drive
Chicago, Illinois 60616-2477
(312) 567-6700

This institute runs a cardiac risk modification program that integrates Western medical practice with behavioral therapy in order to reduce blood pressure, cholesterol levels, and control diabetes. Mind and body techniques are taught to patients by an interdisciplinary staff.

Preventive Medicine Research Institute
900 Bridgeway, Suite 2
Sausalito, California 94965
(415) 332-2525

This organization, founded by Dr. Dean Ornish, offers training programs and conducts research in mind-body medicine.

Cardiac Rehabilitation

Cardiac Rehabilitation
A.H.C.P.R. Publications Clearinghouse
P.O. Box 8547
Silver Spring, Maryland 20907
(800) 358-9295

This pamphlet will give you guidelines for cardiac rehabilitation programs.

Stress and Heart Disease

Stress Reduction Clinic/Department of Medicine
University of Massachusetts Medical Center
55 Lake Avenue North
Worcester, Massachusetts 01655-0267
(508) 856-1616

This outpatient clinic offers an eight-week course for those with a chronic or acute medical conditions. Mindfulness meditation and hatha yoga are taught as the tools to allow the patient to control his or her stress.

TM TRAINING AND STRESS MANAGEMENT COURSES

Your local community college probably offers several different stress reduction and/or meditation programs. Most offer a ten-week beginner course so that you can see how you like it and what benefits it offers.

Smoking

Smoke-Enders
4455 East Camelback Road, Suite D150
Phoenix, Arizona 85018
1-800-828-4357

One of the most reputable smoking-cessation programs in the country, Smoke-Enders has helped countless numbers of addicted smokers to stop. If you call the number above, you'll be referred to a seminar in your local area and begun on a self-start home program that uses tapes, workbooks, and the twenty-four-hour helpline.

American Lung Association
1740 Broadway
New York, New York 10019-4374
1-800-LUNG USA

This organization is dedicated to education, community service, advocacy, and research. When you call, you'll be directed to a local chapter in your area that runs smoking-cessation clinics.

Acupuncture and Chinese Medicine

Council of Colleges of Acupuncture and Oriental Medicine.

8403 Colesville Road, Suite 370
Silver Spring, Maryland 20910
(301) 608-9175

This council will refer you to a traditional Chinese medical practitioner or school of Oriental medicine near you.

National Commission on the Certification of Acupuncture
1424 16th Street NW, Suite 501
Washington, D.C. 20036
(202) 232-1404

This organization offers information on professional standards and licensing requirements for acupuncturists.

American Association of Acupuncture and Oriental Medicine
(address same as above)
(202) 265-2287

This group, which shares the same offices, will give you referrals to practitioners.

Ayurveda

If you wish to find an Ayurvedic practitioner, you may call one of the Maharishi Ayurveda Health Centers around the country. The number to call for a referral is (515) 472-5866.

Biofeedback

American Association of Biofeedback Clinicians
2424 South Demptster Avenue
Des Plaines, Illinois 60016
(312) 827-0440

This organization offers referrals to biofeedback practitioners, hospitals, and pain management centers.

Reflexology

Reflexology Research Project
P.O. Box 35820, Suite D
Albuquerque, New Mexico 87176

This organization can give you information on where to study reflexology or find a reflexologist. They publish a bimonthly newsletter called *Reflexions,* which costs $12.50 a year.

Reiki

The Center for Reiki Training
29209 Northwestern Highway #592
Southfield, Minnesota 48034
1-800-332-8112

This organization can give you information on the location of Reiki masters with whom you can train or receive therapy. They also put out an instructional tape that will take you through first- and second-degree training. They publish a quarterly newsletter, *Reiki News*, available for $5 a year.

Ingredients for Good Heart Health: Where to Order Supplies or Find Referrals

Mail-Order Essence Companies (Aromatherapy)

Aroma Vera
5901 Rodeo Road
Los Angeles, California 90016
1-800-669-9514

Simplers Botanical
P.O. Box 39
Forestville, California 95436
(707) 887-2012

Mail-Order Vitamin Companies

Bronson
P.O. Box 46903
Saint Louis, Missouri 63146-6903
1-800-235-3200

Eclectic Institute
14385 Lusted Road
Sandy, Oregon 97055
1-800-332-HERB

NF Formulas
9775 Southwest Commerce Circle
Wilsonville, Oregon 97070
1-800-547-4891

Thorne Research
P.O. Box 3200
Sandpoint, Idaho 83864
1-800 228-1966

Tyler Encapsulations
2204-8 NW Birdsdale
Gresham, Oregon 97030
(503) 661-5401

L&H Vitamins
37-10 Crescent St.
Long Island City, New York 11101
1-800-221-1152

Mail-Order Homeopathic Remedies

Boiron-Borneman
1204 Amosland Rd.
Norwood, Pennsylvania 19074
1-800 BLU-TUBE

Dolisos
3014 Rigel Ave.
Las Vegas, Nevada 89102
1-800-DOLISOS

Standard Homeopathics
retail brand name is Hyland
Los Angeles, California
1-800 624-9659

Mail-Order Herb Companies

Herb Pharm
P.O. Box 116-N
Williams, Oregon 97544
1-800-348-4372

Herbs of Grace
Division of School of Natural Medicine
P.O. Box 7369
Boulder, Colorado 80306-7369
(303) 443-4882

Herbalist & Alchemist, Inc.
P.O. Box 553
Broadway, New Jersey 08808
(908) 689-9020

Earth's Harvest
2557 Northwest Division
Gresham, Oregon 97030
1-800-428-3308

Nature's Way Products, Inc.
10 Mt. Springs Pkway
Springville, Utah 84663
  (dried herbs, tinctures, capsulated herbs)

Wild Weeds (dried herbs and herbal products)
P.O. Box 88
Redway, California 95560

International Traditional Medicines (Chinese herbs)
Portland, Oregon
(1-800) 544-7504

Eclectic Institute
14385 Lusted Rd.
Sandy, Oregon 97055
1-800-332-HERB

NF Formulas
9775 SW Commerce Circle
Wilsonville, Oregon 97070
1-800 547-4891

Chinese Herbs
International Traditional Medicines (Chinese herbs)
2017 Southeast Hawthorn
Portland, Oregon 97214
1-800-544-7504

East Earth Trade Winds
P.O. Box 493151
Redding, California 96049-3151
1-800-258-6878

Nuherbs Company
3820 Penniman Avenue
Oakland, California 94619
1-800-233-4307

These companies have a full catalog of Chinese herbs, books, and supplements.

Ayurvedic Products

The various oils, herbs, raw-silk gloves for massage, and other Ayurvedic products are available from

Maharishi Ayurveda Products International, Inc.
P.O. Box 541
Lancaster, Massachusetts 01523
1-800-255-8332
(508) 368-8101 (Massachusetts, Alaska, and Hawaii)

Available Libraries and Databases

If you're on-line with any computer network such as Medline or Paperchase on CompuServe, you can look up articles from medical libraries all over the country—including scientific journals that cover alternative health care.

You may also wish to contact the groups listed below:

Center for Medical Consumers/Health Care Library
237 Thompson Street

New York, New York 10012
(212) 674-7105

This is an excellent resource for books and the latest articles on conventional and alternative medicine. They also publish a monthly newsletter called *Healthfacts*.

World Research Foundation
15300 Ventura Boulevard, Suite 405
Sherman Oaks, California 91403
(818) 907-5483

This organization provides information packs on health subjects. For a fee of $45 plus shipping they will research either standard or alternative medical approaches to any disease or condition, calling on information from five thousand medical journal articles and a variety of books on complementary treatments.

Planetree Health Resource Center
2040 Webster Street
San Francisco, California 94115
(415) 923-3681

Planetree offers an In-Depth Information Packet for $100 that offers a selection of up-to-date medical references, or you can order a $20 bibliography of source materials. They can also supply you with their directory of physicians and other health care practitioners, organizations, and support groups.

The Health Resource
Janice R. Guthrie
209 Katerine Drive
Conway, Arizona 72032
(501) 329-5272

They will provide reports on traditional and alternative treatments of specific medical problems for a fee of $195 plus shipping.

Hot Line

Heartlife (1-800-241-6993); or, in Alaska or Georgia, call collect (404) 523-0826. Information on heart disease, pacemakers, nutrition, and medication.

Recommended Reading

Newsletters
Diet-Heart Newsletter
P.O. Box 2039
Venice, California 90294

This costs $15 a year and is published quarterly by health book author Robert Kowalski, including recipes and nutritional information.

Heartline
Cleveland Clinic Educational Foundation
Coronary Club, Inc.
9500 Euclid Avenue, E4-15
Cleveland, Ohio 44195-5058
This costs $29 a year for twelve issues.

Cooking for Your Heart
In order to keep your heart in the best shape, you have to eat right. Here are some recommended heart-healthy cookbooks:

The American Heart Association Cookbook, 4th revised edition (David McKay Co., New York, 1986).

Claiborne, Craig. *Craig Claiborne's Gourmet Diet* (Ballantine Books, New York, 1985).

Connor, Sonja J., M.S., R.D.; and William Connor, M.D. *The New American Diet* (Simon & Schuster, New York, 1989).

Longbotham, Lori, *Quick and Easy Recipes to Lower Your Cholesterol* (Avon Books, New York, 1989).

Piscatilla, Joseph, *Don't Eat Your Heart Out Cookbook* (Workman Publishing Co., Inc., New York, 1983).

Books

Austin, Phyllis; and Agatha M. Thrash, *Natural Remedies: A Manual* (NewLife Books, Santa Cruz, Calif., 1983).

———, *More Natural Remedies* (NewLife Books, 1984).

Balch, James F., M.D.; and Phyllis A. Balch, C.N.C., *Prescription for Nutritional Healing* (Avery Publishing Group, Inc., Garden City Park, N.Y., 1990).

Beinfield, Harriet, L.Ac. and Etrem Korngold, L.Ac., O.M.J. *Between Heaven and Earth: A Guide to Chinese Medicine* (Ballantine Books, New York, 1991).

Benson, Herbert, *The Relaxation Response* (William Morrow and Co., New York, 1975).

Borland, Douglas, M.D., *Homeopathy in Practice* (Keats Publishing, New Canaan, Conn., 1982).

Boyd, Hamish, W., M.D., *Introduction to Homeopathic Medicine* (Keats Publishing, Inc., New Canaan, Conn., 1981).

Buchman, Dian Dincin, *Herbal Medicine: The Natural Way to Get Well and Stay Well* (Gramercy Publishing Co., New York, 1980).

Burton Goldberg Group, *Alternative Medicine: The Definitive Guide* (Future Medicine Publishing, Puyallup, Wash.: 1993).

Chopra, Deepak, M.D., *Perfect Health* (Bantam Books, New York, 1990).

Dossey, Larry, *Healing Words* (Bantam Books, New York, 1994).

Gash, Michael Reed, *Acupressure's Potent Points* (Bantam Books, New York, 1990).

Hoffmann, David, *The Holistic Herbal* (Healing Arts Press, Rochester, Vt., 1990).

Horan, Paula, *Empowerment Through Reiki* (Lotus Light/ Shangri-La, Wilmot, Wisc., 1992).

Kabat-Zinn, Jon, *Full Catastrophe Living* (Delta Books, New York, 1990).

———, *Wherever You Go, There You Are* (Hyperion Books, New York, 1994).

Kaptchuk, Ted, O.M.D., *The Web That Has No Weaver: Understanding Chinese Medicine* (Congdon & Weed, New York, 1983).

Krochmal, Arnold and Connie, *A Field Guide to Medicinal Plants* (Times Books, New York, 1973, 1984).

Lowen, Alexander, M.D., *Love, Sex and Your Heart: The Health-Happiness Connection* (Penguin USA, New York, 1988).

Lynch, J. J., *The Broken Heart* (Basic Books, New York, 1977).

———, *The Language of the Heart: The Body's Response to Human Dialogue* (Basic Books, New York, 1985).

Mabey, Richard, *The New Age Herbalist* (Collier Books, Macmillan Publishing Co., New York, 1988).

Mindell, Earl, *Earl Mindell's Herb Bible* (Fireside/Simon & Schuster, New York, 1992.

Mowrey, Daniel B., Ph.D., *The Scientific Validation of Herbal Medicine* (Keats Publishing, Inc., New Canaan, Conn., 1986).

Murray, Michael T., N.D., and Joseph E. Pizzorno, N.D. *An Encyclopedia of Natural Medicine* (Prima Publishing, Rocklin, Calif., 1991).

Olshelvsky, Moshe, et al., *Manual of Natural Therapy* (Facts on File, New York, 1989).

Ornish, Dean, M.D., *Dr. Dean Ornish's Program for Reversing Heart Disease* (Random House, New York, 1990).

————, *Stress, Diet and Your Heart* (Holt, Rinehart & Winston, New York, 1982).

Panos, Maesimund B.; and Jane Heimlich, *Homeopathic Medicine at Home* (J.P. Tarcher, Inc., Los Angeles, 1980).

People's Medical Society, *Your Heart: Questions You Have, Answers You Need* (People's Medical Society, Allentown, Pa., 1992).

Robertson, Laurel, *Laurel's Kitchen Recipes* (Ten Speed Press, New York, 1993).

Ross, Elizabeth, M.D., F.A.C.C.; and Judith Sachs, *Healing the Female Heart* (Pocket Books, New York, 1995).

Roth, Eli, M., M.D., F.A.C.C.; and Sandra L. Streicher, R.N., *Good Cholesterol, Bad Cholesterol* (Prima Publishing and Communications, Rocklin, Calif., 1990).

Simon, Harvey B., M.D., *Conquering Heart Disease: New Ways to Live Well Without Drugs or Surgery* (Little, Brown & Co., 1994).

Thomas, Richard, *The Natural Way with Heart Disease* (Element Press, Rockport, Mass., 1994).

Tisserand, Robert, *Aromatherapy* (Healing Arts Press, Rochester, Vt., 1985, 1988).

Ullman, Dana, *Discovering Homeopathy* (North Atlantic Books, Berkeley, Calif., 1988, 1991).

Wade, Carlson, *Inner Cleansing: How to Free Yourself from Joint-Muscle-Artery-Circulation Sludge* (Parker Publishing Company, West Nyack, N.Y., 1992).

Weed, Susun S., *Healing Wise* (Ash Tree Publishing, Woodstock, N.Y., 1989).

Weil, Andrew, M.D., *Natural Health, Natural Medicine* (Houghton, Mifflin Co. Boston, 1990).

Werbach, Melvyn R., M.D., *Nutritional Influences on Illness* (Third Line Press, Inc., Tarzana, Calif., 1987, 1988).

Wolfe, Honora Lee, *Second Spring: A Guide to Healthy Menopause Through Traditional Chinese Medicine* (Blue Poppy Press, Boulder, Colo., 1992).

Zhou, Dahong, M.D., *The Chinese Exercise Book* (Hartley & Marks, Pt. Roberts, Wash., 1984).

Glossary

Acupoints: The various points along any meridian that can be stimulated in order to achieve healing. (See *acupuncture*)

Acupuncture: A system of Chinese medicine that uses fine stainless steel needles to access energy along any one of the body's pathways, or meridians.

Aerobic activity: Vigorous exercise that raises the heart rate by at least 70 percent of its maximum capacity and keeps it there for at least twenty minutes.

Alexander technique: A movement system developed by a nineteenth-century actor that restores function and alignment to the body.

Allopathic medicine: The traditional Western practice of medicine, which is based on curing illness.

Angina: Severe pain and constriction around the heart related to an insufficient supply of blood to the heart.

Angiogram (or **arteriogram**): The gold standard of allopathic cardiac diagnosis where a catheter is snaked into the heart to determine the amount of blockage in the coronary arteries.

Angioplasty (also known as PTCA): An invasive procedure where a small balloon is introduced by a catheter into the heart to expand a blocked artery.

Antioxidant: Protective enzymes, amino acids, vitamins and minerals, and other compounds that act as scavengers in the body to eliminate free radicals.

Aromatherapy: Herbal therapy using the essential oil of certain plants, which are inhaled or rubbed on the body during a massage.

Arrhythmia: Any interruption in the heart's rhythm. An arrhythmia may consist of a missed beat, skipped beats, or abnormal beats.

Arterial spasm: A "cramp" or torquing inside an artery that causes exquisite pain but is not always evident on an electrocardiogram.

Atherosclerosis (also known as coronary artery disease, or CAD): Caused by a loss of oxygen and nutrients to the heart muscle because of diminished blood flow. In this disease, plaque collects on the inside of arterial walls, narrowing and eventually obstructing the flow of blood and possibly leading to a heart attack or stroke.

Atrium: One of the top two chambers of the heart. The right atrium receives unoxygenated blood returning from the veins; the left atrium receives oxygenated blood from the lungs and delivers it to the left ventricle.

Ayurveda: "The science of prolonged life." The ancient Indian system of healing based on preventive care and a philosophy of good living that is specific to each individual.

Beta-endorphins: Neurotransmitters that give us a sense of well-being and that are released when we relax or are positively stimulated.

Biofeedback: A method of learning to monitor your body processes and alter them based on feedback from a machine.

Bypass surgery: An invasive procedure where a vein is taken from the leg or chest and attached to the heart to divert blood flow past the blockage in an artery.

Caffeine: A nervous system stimulant found in coffee, tea, cocoa, chocolate, and soda. It appears to raise cholesterol levels and to create irregular heartbeats in some individuals.

Cardiotonic: Having the ability to make the heart pump more efficiently.

Chelation: A system of washing the insides of arteries via an intravenous drip of vitamins, amino acids, and minerals that bind to metals and flush them out of your system.

Chinese or Oriental medicine: The ancient system of healing based on the balance of *yin* and *yang* as well as the five elements of Water, Wood, Fire, Earth, and Metal.

Cholesterol: A waxlike substance created in the body by the liver and also consumed along with dietary fat. There are two types of cholesterol: the LDLs, which help plaque to form on your arteries; and the HDLs, which keep plaque off the arteries.

Congestive heart failure: A condition that results when the left ventricle cannot pump the amount of blood the body needs. Symptoms include shortness of breath, palpitations, and great fatigue. This condition can affect other organs and may predispose one to a shortened life span.

Coronary arteries: The three arteries (and a fourth, which branches off) that encircle the heart like a crown and give it its own blood supply.

Coronary artery disease: See *atherosclerosis.*

Cyanotic: Blue-colored. A sign that the body is not getting enough oxygenated blood.

Decoction: An infusion reduced by evaporation, therefore four to sixteen times more potent.

Diabetes: A disorder of blood sugar regulation caused by the body's inability to use insulin appropriately. This condition may predispose one to heart disease and other illnesses.

Diaphoretic: Sweat-inducing.

Dis-stress: Negative stress caused by too much or too little arousal, which disrupts body and mind.

Diuretic: A drug or other substance that removes water and salt from the body so that blood volume goes up and the heart doesn't have to work as hard.

Dosha: One of three body and personality types in Ayurveda.

Edema: Swelling.

Energetic therapies: Healing arts that use the energy of the body (as opposed to the biology or chemistry of the body) to heal itself. Homeopathy, Reiki, and reflexology are such therapies.

Eu-stress: Good stress, the type that challenges you.

Feldenkrais: A movement system developed by an Israeli scientist designed to release habitual patterns of tension in the body.

Fiber: The indigestible cell-wall material of plants, found to enhance the cholesterol-lowering effects of a low-fat diet.

Fibrillation: When the walls of the chambers of the heart contract in a rapid, nonrhythmic beat. Atrial fibrillation (as many as three hundred beats a minute) often occurs after a heart attack, but is usually not life-threatening; ventricular fibrillation prevents blood from flowing to the rest of the body and may result in death.

"Fight or flight": The immediate physical reaction of the body to stress as the stress hormones are released. This causes clammy hands, heart palpitations, headache, and a knot in the stomach.

Flavonoids: Colored aromatic substances found in plants that have healing properties.

Free radicals: Wild chemical reactants that assist in the destructive process of oxidation in a cell. Free radicals are partly responsible for the formation of plaque on arteries.

HDLs: High-density lipoproteins, the "good" cholesterol that keeps plaque off the arteries.

Herbal medicine: The science of using herbs' medicinal properties for healing.

Holistic medicine: The practice of treating the whole individual—body, mind, and spirit—to enhance wellness rather than isolating one organ or tissue in order to cure disease.

Homeopathy: The treatment that uses the body's energy to heal itself. The theory behind homeopathy is that "like cures like," or a little bit of something that might make a well person ill will help to heal a sick person. By dosing the individual with remedies that mimic the symptoms of heart disease, the body is able to rally its own energies and fight the disease.

Homocysteine (HCY): A toxic amino acid that causes arterial lesions.

Hypercholesterolemia: The condition of having an abnormally high cholesterol level.

Hypertension: High blood pressure, classified as anything above 140/90.

Hypothalamus: The master "switch-on" gland for the body, which sends messages to all other glands. The hypothalamus is also responsible for the body's temperature, metabolism, emotional regulation, and other vital functions.

Infusion: A mixture of herbs that has been covered with boiling water and allowed to steep. The ratio is one ounce of herb to a pint of water.

Ischemia: Reduced blood flow to the heart.

Isometric activity: Strength exercises such as weight training, where you lift while the body is static.

Jing: In Chinese medicine, it is believed to be the source of our ability to reproduce and develop properly.

LDLs: Low-density lipoproteins, the "bad" cholesterol that allows plaque to accumulate on the arterial walls.

Legume: A group of foods with a vegetable protein base, such as peas and beans.

Meditation: The practice of calming the mind through breath and relaxation techniques.

Meridians: The Chinese "pathways" through the energy systems of the body. There are twelve meridians, connected by a series of acupoints.

Mindfulness: A type of meditation where you concentrate fully and completely on the activity you are doing, whether it is brushing your teeth or climbing a mountain.

Mineral: An inorganic substance that remains after living plant or animal tissue is burned off. Minerals work in conjunction with enzymes, hormones, and vitamins and help in a variety of body processes.

Mitral valve prolapse: A condition, common in women, where the mitral valve becomes enlarged and floppy and doesn't snap shut, allowing blood to seep backward into the atrium. This causes a "click" sound on examination.

Myocardial infarction: Heart attack.

Neurotransmitters: Substances that are released when a neuron is excited. They act as the "hormones" of the central nervous system, sending emotional messages throughout the body, telling us how to react to various situations.

Occlusion: Blockage. Where plaque has completely blocked an artery leading to the heart.

Omega-3 fatty acids: Beneficial fats found in cold-water fish and some quasi-vitamins.

Palpitations: Rapid, pounding heartbeats.

Parasympathetic nervous system: The portion of the autonomic nervous system that triggers the "relaxation response" so that our mind and body can return to normal after being stressed.

Plaque: Sometimes called atheromatous plaque. The accumulation of fat and waste on the inside of the arterial wall, most prevalent in individuals who consume a high-fat, high-cholesterol diet with no exercise and high stress. Plaque eventually solidifies and makes it difficult for blood to flow through.

Platelets: A part of the blood responsible for clotting.

Potentiation: The process of diluting a homeopathic remedy (either of plant, mineral, or animal origin) in water or alcohol so that only the "phantom" of the original substance exists.

Primordial sounds: Vibrations that balance the body, which can be used in meditation, such as the sound *Om*.

qi (sometimes spelled "chi" or "ki"): Energy, life force.

qi gong (sometimes spelled "chi gung"): Breathwork, a Chinese healing art used for prevention and treatment of chronic disease.

RDA: Required Daily Allowances, the amount of vitamins and minerals necessary to avoid deficiencies, set by the Food and Drug Administration.

Reflexology: The practice of massaging and stimulating specific areas of the foot that correspond to other parts of the body.

Reiki: It means "universal transcendent spirit" and is a Japanese form of touch therapy that channels energy for healing throughout the body.

Relaxation response: A term coined by Dr. Herbert Benson, referring to the action of the parasympathetic nervous system, which returns heart rate to normal, restores peripheral blood flow, reduces respiration, and so on.

Saturated fat: A fat that is solid at room temperature, such as butter, lard, and animal fat. It raises LDLs and also stimulates the liver to produce cholesterol.

Shen: In Chinese medicine, the attribute of spirit or aliveness.

Soy protein: Protein found in soybeans or products made from them, such as tofu, tempeh, and miso, and found to cut cholesterol dramatically when consumed in amounts exceeding 47 grams daily.

Stress: Any stimulus created by ourselves, others, or the environment that causes normal bodily functions to be disrupted. Our perception of an event as difficult or unsettling.

Stress hormones: Adrenaline, noradrenaline, and cortisol, the adrenal hormones released when we experience the "fight or flight" response and our sympathetic nervous system is activated.

Stroke: A condition that occurs when blood flow cannot reach the brain. A stroke may be caused by a plaque breaking off and traveling to the brain, or by a ruptured blood vessel in the brain.

Succussion: The process of shaking a homeopathic remedy in order to activate the energy inherent in it.

Supplementation: Adding vitamins, minerals, and quasi-vitamins in pill or powder form to one's diet.

Sympathetic nervous system: The first reactor of the autonomic nervous system, telling the body that it must be on red alert. When aroused, this system triggers the stress hormones and creates clammy hands, palpitations, a knot in the stomach, tension headaches.

Tachycardia: Heart palpitations; quick, pounding heartbeats.

Tai chi chuan: Translates as "grand ultimate fist." The Chinese system of moving meditation that integrates mind and body. It involves practicing forms or choreographed patterns of movement that activate various acupoints and stimulate the internal organs.

T-cells: Cells produced by the immune system to help the body heal.

Tincture (sometimes called **extract**): A way of preparing herbs by soaking them in a mixture of alcohol and water to cull the most potent substances from them.

Triglycerides: A damaging form of fat, carried in VLDLs (very-low-density lipoproteins.) Elevated levels are common in coronary artery disease.

Unsaturated fat: Fats that are not naturally solid at room temperature. The good ones (monounsaturated) will reduce LDLs and leave HDLs intact. The bad ones (polyunsaturated) have been partially hydrogenated so that they will stand up on bread and produce trans-fatty acids that raise LDLs and lower HDLs.

Valve: The opening from atria to ventricle; a one-way mechanism for blood to flow through the heart.

Vasodilator: Any substance (medication, herb, remedy) that causes blood vessels to dilate.

Ventricle: One of the two lower chambers of the heart. The right ventricle pumps blood into the lungs so that it can be oxygenated; the left ventricle pumps blood out to the rest of the body through the arteries.

Visualization: Sometimes known as guided imagery. The practice of imagining a positive scene and putting yourself into it in order to evoke a feeling of relaxation.

Vitamin: An organic substance that cannot be synthesized in the body and must be ingested in the diet or by supplementation. There are two varieties, water-soluble and fat-soluble.

Yin/yang: The two opposite principles that combine to create one whole in Chinese philosophy. The *yin* is the receptive, yielding capacity within us; the *yang* is the strong and untiring capacity. All things in the universe have some *yin* and *yang* within them, and it is by keeping them in balance that we remain healthy.

Yoga: An ancient Indian series of postures combined with breathing that unifies mind and body, using mental power to generate internal and external healing. Daily yoga practice will lower blood pressure and heart rate.

Zone therapy: The guiding principle of reflexology, which states that the body is divided into ten longitudinal zones that encompass all the organs.

INDEX

About the Author

Judith Sachs, the daughter and granddaughter of physicians, was born in New York City. A health and medical writer and speaker, she is the co-author of *Healing the Female Heart* (Pocket Books) with Dr. Elizabeth Ross and is the author of *The Healing Power of Sex* (Prentice Hall/Paramount Publishing), *What Women Should Know About Menopause, What You Can Do About Osteoporosis* (Dell Medical Library Series), and thirteen other books on preventive health care.

Judith Sachs conducts workshops and seminars at holistic centers, corporations, and universities and has lectured extensively on subjects from midlife and longevity to parenting and HIV/AIDS prevention. She has served as an adjunct professor at Trenton State College in the stress management program.

The author lives in central New Jersey with her husband and daughter and is currently working on a book about natural remedies for mental and emotional problems.